# WORKING WITH
# FAMILY CARERS

EARLY
INTERVENTION,
PREVENTION
& SUPPORT

**Other books you may be interested in:**

*Active Social Work with Children with Disabilities*
By Julie Adams and Diana Leshone
ISBN 978-1-910391-94-5

*Anti-Racism in Social Work Practice*
Edited by Angie Bartoli
ISBN 978-1-909330-13-9

*The Critical Years: Child Development from Conception to Five*
By Tim Gully
ISBN 978-1-909330-73-3

*Evidencing CPD – A Guide to Building Your Social Work Portfolio*
By Daisy Bogg and Maggie Challis
ISBN 978-1-909330-25-2

*Mental Health and the Criminal Justice System*
By Ian Cummins
ISBN 978-1-910391-90-7

*Modern Mental Health: Critical Perspectives on Psychiatric Practice*
Edited by Steven Walker
ISBN 978-1-909330-53-5

*Observing Children and Families: Beyond the Surface*
By Gill Butler
ISBN 978-1-910391-62-4

*Personal Safety for Social Workers and Health Professionals*
By Brian Atkins
ISBN 978-1-909330-33-7

*Positive Social Work: The Essential Toolkit for NQSWs*
By Julie Adams and Angie Sheard
ISBN 978-1-909330-05-4

*Practice Education in Social Work: Achieving Professional Standards*
By Pam Field, Cathie Jasper and Lesley Littler
ISBN 978-1-909330-17-7

*Psychosocial and Relationship-Based Practice*
By Claudia Megele
ISBN 978-1-909682-97-9

*Self-Neglect: A Practical Approach to Risks and Strengths Assessment*
By Shona Britten and Karen Whitby
ISBN 978-1-912096-86-2

*The Social Worker's Guide to the Care Act*
By Pete Feldon
ISBN 978-1-911106-68-5

*Starting Social Work: Reflections of a Newly Qualified Social Worker*
By Rebecca Joy Novell
ISBN 978-1-909682-09-2

*Understanding Substance Use: Policy and Practice*
By Elaine Arnull
ISBN 978-1-909330-93-1

*What's Your Problem? Making Sense of Social Policy and the Policy Process*
By Stuart Connor
ISBN 978-1-909330-49-8

Titles are also available in a range of electronic formats. To order please go to our website www.criticalpublishing.com or contact our distributor NBN International, 10 Thornbury Road, Plymouth PL6 7PP, telephone 01752 202301 or email orders@nbninternational.com

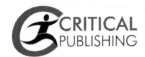
CRITICAL
PUBLISHING

# WORKING WITH
# FAMILY CARERS

Valerie Gant

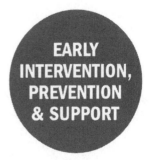
EARLY
INTERVENTION,
PREVENTION
& SUPPORT

First published in 2018 by Critical Publishing Ltd

British Library Cataloguing in Publication Data
A CIP record for this book is available from the British Library

ISBN: 978-1-912096-97-8

This book is also available in the following e-book formats:
MOBI ISBN: 978-1-912096-96-1
EPUB ISBN: 978-1-912096-95-4
Adobe e-book ISBN: 978-1-912096-94-7

Cover design by Out of House
Text design by Greensplash Limited
Project management by Out of House Publishing
Printed and bound in Great Britain by 4edge, Essex

Critical Publishing
3 Connaught Road
St Albans
AL3 5RX

www.criticalpublishing.com

Paper from responsible sources

# Acknowledgments and dedication

In writing this book I would like to acknowledge the following:

My family and friends for listening to my ideas and encouraging me, most especially Paula and Steve.

Colleagues and students at the University of Chester, especially Eve Collins and Mandy Schofield.

Family carers everywhere – you can do this and you can do it well.

Lastly, I wish to dedicate this book to my youngest daughter who has taught me more about caring than any textbook in the world could ever do.

Isobel – this is for you.

# Contents

*Meet the author and series editor*       *viii*

*Series editor foreword*       *ix*

Chapter 1    Introduction: Why this book and why now?       1

Chapter 2    Background to informal care       19

Chapter 3    Law, policy, politics and people       41

Chapter 4    Carers: Caring and care-giving       64

Chapter 5    Professionals and caring       85

Chapter 6    Research and practice       108

Chapter 7    Young carers, older parent-carers and carers of people with dementia       130

Chapter 8    Reflections and conclusion: Looking to the future       152

*Index*       *173*

# Dr Valerie Gant (author)

Dr Valerie Gant is an experienced social work practitioner and senior lecturer at the University of Chester. Val has written and published on a variety of subjects relating to health and social care. Her personal experience of having a child with severe learning difficulties has both inspired and informed her in-depth professional knowledge of this area. An active researcher, Val is interested in carers, disability issues and auto-ethnography, both as a process and as a method, and has recently published a paper on this method in the journal *Qualitative Social Work* (*QSW*).

She lives by the sea, and when she isn't writing and researching she enjoys walking her dog and spending time with her family.

# Dr Steve J Hothersall (series editor)

Dr Steve J Hothersall is the Head of Social Work Education at Edge Hill University and both a registered social worker and a registered nurse. He has written on social work practice with children, young people and their families, mental health, need, social policy and philosophy, especially epistemology. Steve has also served on the Editorial Board of the *British Journal of Social Work* and reviews for a range of academic journals. His academic interests relate to methodology, the use of philosophy to inform both teaching and practice, and research focusing on the development and use of professional knowledge, drawing on underpinning epistemic principles and considering their role and application in knowledge communities. He is currently working on developing and implementing a model to support practice and research underpinned by reference to philosophical pragmatism. He is also passionate about the music of Ludwig van Beethoven, and the role of music in the promotion of wellbeing.

# Series editor foreword

It is with great pleasure that I write this foreword for the first book in what is hoped will be a noteworthy and innovative series for Critical Publishing entitled 'Early Intervention, Prevention and Support'. Val Gant's 'Working with Family Carers' is perhaps a particularly noteworthy title, as its focus epitomises what this triad aims to focus upon. Family (and informal) carers are perhaps the frontline in terms of early intervention, prevention and support, so to launch this series with such a well-crafted text is apposite.

Val is a senior lecturer in social work at the University of Chester, based at the Warrington campus, and brings many years of practical, professional and *personal* experience to her writing. This topic is one very close to Val, both personally and professionally, as even a cursory glance at the text will reveal, and what is particularly revealing is the way in which the writing utilises both perspectives to the fullest extent.

The book sets out to explain the myriad complex realities of being a family/informal carer, juxtaposing these with the contemporary nature of professional social work practice. Within its pages, we are introduced to the contemporary nature of family and informal caring, with new statutory provisions being highlighted to contextualise the prevailing landscape. Definitions of core concepts are provided and the reader is introduced to the 'world' of family and informal caring, aided by the effective and creative use of case studies and exercises. Along the way there are chapters that focus on the background to informal care, revealing how and why things are the way they are today, highlighting the gendered nature of care and its economic implications, for the government, and for all of us. There is detailed commentary on the legal and policy content, and careful and empathetic consideration of what it is, and must be like, to be a family/informal carer, and the impact that can have on people, in both good and not-so-good ways. Chapters on the role of professionals in this domain are given equally effective treatment, thus allowing practitioners from a range of different professions and occupations the opportunity to reflect deeply on what they do and how they do it, for good, or for ill. The text also considers relevant research that has helped guide and inform the current care landscape, and a special focus is given to young carers, older parent-carers and those caring for those with dementia and similar conditions, before the final chapter asks us to reflect and look to the future.

This is a book that draws on the author's professional, personal and human experiences of care and care-giving, and as such offers what I perceive as a profoundly moral perspective. In its pages we can begin to understand that many people's lives are dedicated to the wellbeing of others, often at the expense of their own wellbeing. That this happens all day, and every day for some is, quite frankly, not only revelatory, but shocking. The dilemmas inherent within such mundane, everyday tasks as helping someone to dress themselves are revealed in full technicolour, and challenge us all – as professionals, policy makers and the public, to rethink the role of family and informal carers in different ways, and re-evaluate how we manage and support, holistically and structurally, what is a truly herculean task.

Family and informal carers are not only at the frontline of caring for those who are vulnerable, but they are the frontline. Professional services, be they state-sponsored or part of the private, voluntary and independent sector would be decimated overnight if family and informal carers were provided with the support they require at the level they actually require it. It is perhaps not understating it to say that those professional support services, well-intentioned as they are, and its workers, well-motivated as they are, are only really touching the sides of something so pervasive and enormous, that to err in supporting this task is to risk many people and their communities imploding, with dire consequences for us all.

This text is pivotal – not only as the first in a new series, but as a text in its own right, on a topic given much less academic, professional and governmental attention than it truly deserves. I have been moved and inspired by some of the insights afforded to me by reading Val's work – and I believe that this book will do much to invigorate this topic – and focus necessary attention on an issue that is likely to affect most, if not all of us at some time in our lives. We owe it not only to family and informal carers, but to ourselves, to take seriously the issues this book raises, and to respond appropriately. And therein lies a challenge to the ways in which we currently configure our support of family and informal carers, a challenge that the government should heed.

Dr Steve J Hothersall, Series Editor
Head of Social Work Education, Edge Hill

# Chapter 1 | Introduction: Why this book and why now?

Over the last three decades, the titles 'care-giver' and 'carer', as both a role and as socially recognised and (perhaps) accepted 'entities' have emerged. Changes in legislation which enshrine such recognition have now occurred, most recently in the Care Act (2014) which arrived with much promise and potential for optimism, with politicians going so far as to proclaim it *'[T]he most significant reform of care and support for 60 years'* (Lamb, 2014).

Demographic changes in society, an increase in life expectancy – seen as a celebration in the twentieth century, and a challenge in the twenty-first century (Macnicol, 2015) – as well as policies aimed at supporting this group of people, many of whom have illnesses associated with age, all add to the realisation of the ubiquitous existence of carers and of them having a definable role. Although there has been a growth in total life expectancy, this has been outpaced by the issues associated with the number of older people who are frail and living with co-morbidities (Hulme et al, 2016). Due, therefore, to the increasing health and social care needs of an older population, the likelihood of people needing a high level of intensive support as they age has increased. The effect of the pressures on health and social care brought about by the current economic climate also has an impact on the likelihood of an individual needing 'informal' care. National health and social care services now only tend to work with those in crisis, and on a short-term basis, meaning friends and relatives support and assist with care that in decades past would more likely have been addressed within the 'professional' arena. According to the 2011 Census, 10.3 per cent of the UK population provided unpaid care (ONS, 2013), an increase of 600,000 since the 2001 Census, the first time a question on the provision of unpaid care was asked, and this number looks set to increase, with the most intense caring, that of over 50 hours a week, increasing most (Carers UK, 2015; Franklin, 2015; Robards et al, 2015).

As well as the issue of physical decline, there is a notable increase in the number of people recorded as having dementia and associated mental health impairments (Alzheimer's Association, 2017; de Boer et al, 2015). Put simply, people are living longer, but the older one is, the more likely one is to be in poorer health and in receipt of care, most likely 'informal', ie unpaid care from friends or relatives. The emotional and psychological challenges of care-giving as well as the practical and physical impact need therefore to be recognised, understood, acknowledged, and supported. For practitioners working with and supporting carers, developing their own understanding of what caring is, and means, may lead to an increase in the building and developing of crucial relationships and may be the key to finding a gateway into that unique situation, culminating in a deeper and more successful connection. I believe it is that connection and our possession of the capacity to empathise that separates us out as a species and offers hope for the future. As professionals, we are duty bound to do the best we can with what we have at our disposal. As human beings, we are morally bound to recognise the importance of caring and to accord it the status it deserves. This text will hopefully provide the basis for a more enlightened and engaged appreciation of one of the most significant roles and functions within society – caring. Offering a discussion and analysis of some of the key research areas related to caring and highlighting these through the use of case study examples, this book offers a way to begin to explore the impact of caring on the lives of family carers and the effectiveness of support, as well as exploring ways to acknowledging this crucial role.

The aim of this introductory chapter is to begin to explore definitions of care and care-giving, and identify the perspective from which it is being considered, as well as providing an overview of the structure of the chapters that follow. The chapter will introduce the reader to the format of the book, designed as it is to encourage interaction: each chapter is designed to be worked through using case study examples and reflective and practical tasks. Further reading is suggested at the end of each chapter and a list of resources will be included.

# Aims of the book

There is an ever-increasing reliance on family carers in everyday life (Carers UK, 2015; Hulme et al, 2016; Smith et al, 2015) with reports regarding the issue regularly appearing in the media; for example: *"Undercover carers' save the taxpayer £40 billion a year'* (Daily Express 15 Dec 2016). *'I became my mother-in-law's carer – but I just couldn't handle the stress of the job'* (Daily Telegraph 5 May 2017) and *'The crisis of young carers: 'Going to school is a break''* (The Guardian 26 Jan 2017). It is a topic also covered widely by radio; for example: Radio 2 'Carers Week' 6 Jun 2016; Radio 4 'The Secret Lives of Carers' 1 Dec 2015, and yet there is surprisingly little clarity regarding what 'caring' and 'care-giving' really means in real, practical terms. From a relatively simple word comes a vague, ambiguous and invariably complex phenomenon, and yet one which many people accept without question and believe they understand. For many, including those who are providing a significant amount of unpaid care to friends and/or relatives, carers are still seen as 'other people', generally provided by social care agencies and importantly 'the ones who are paid'. The implications for (a lack of) identity of carers has significant consequences, and some of the reasons behind this, including the gendered nature of caring, the fact that caring takes place in the private sphere, and that the work undertaken by carers can be messy, unpleasant and hard, is discussed and explored in Chapter 4.

It is important to make the point here that this book is about those 6.5 million *unpaid* 'informal' carers, 1.6 million of whom provide 50 or more hours of care per week (Carers UK, 2015), with no pay, and often little support in managing their day-to-day activities. In the UK it has been estimated that the demand for care brought about by an ageing population will soon outstrip supply (McNeil and Hunter, 2014), and the ways in which carers or care-givers (I will use the terms interchangeably throughout the book) are supported by the state has an impact that goes beyond any individual situation. This book then is about care and care-givers, is intended as a text book for students of social work, social care, those in health care (nurses, occupational therapists, physiotherapists) and other cognate disciplines and as noted above, is written about those whom I call 'family' care-givers: those for whom caring is not a term of specific employment, and for whom there is little recompense. I debated about using the term 'informal' as opposed to 'family' carers; however, for me the term 'informal' does carers something of a disservice, as that term implies that caring is an activity undertaken casually, with some degree of choice in taking on the role, and a lack of responsibility for outcomes associated with the tasks of caring. Such is not the case for many. This book therefore, is for both students and practitioners, designed as a way of helping to work through and make sense of a very complex terrain. While paid carers will also find information of use in this book, the primary focus is on those who provide care for a family member, friend or neighbour in an unpaid capacity.

Recent legislative changes in the UK brought about by the Care Act (2014) have now altered the profile of carers, and as such a text of this nature is timely. The changing demographics of society mentioned above: people living longer and many more living with life-limiting illnesses brought about by the diagnosis and recognition of previously unrecognised disabilities, has increased the need for an up-to-date text that may be used by students and practitioners across the range of health and social care professions.

# A professional and a personal perspective

This book was brought about following several research projects I have carried out exploring the lives of parent-carers of adults with learning disabilities. As a social worker, working in what was at the time a specialised adults with learning disability team, I noted and recognised the impact of care-giving and receiving care on people's lives. It is never a straightforward one-way process, and throughout my career I have observed many examples of reciprocal care. As an educator, working with social work and health and social care undergraduates and post-graduates, I have noted how the involvement of carers is threaded through all the modules and programmes I teach. For example, 'interprofessional working', 'critical social work practice', 'safeguarding vulnerable groups', 'social work law and ethics', as well as research and dissertation modules all engage with carers and the issues they face. Students also bring their own unique experiences of being carers (and in some instances, of receiving care) to the classroom and I have been privileged to listen to the many examples that care-giving students draw on to begin to make sense of their own place within this terrain. Likewise, several colleagues are involved in complex caring scenarios and I have noted and heard anecdotally that some employers are becoming aware of and are seeking ways of supporting staff members with caring responsibilities, beyond those of raising children.

Although this book is written primarily from a professional perspective, it is also my personal experience of being a parent-carer that has had a significant influence and impact on my values, my focus and the overall perspective provided here. My youngest daughter has what is currently referred to as a 'severe learning disability' and at the time of writing this book she is undergoing the transition between children and adult services. The personal experiences I have gained shape and frame my reference point when exploring issues relating to carers and it would be disingenuous of me not to acknowledge this here.

# Definitions

As with many topics and social issues, understanding exactly what it is you are talking and thinking about is quite useful – hence the need to consider definitions. Notions of caring, care and care-giving are, as you might expect, fraught with ambiguity, confusion and misunderstanding. Here we will consider some of these in order that you can begin to appreciate some of the dimensions and complexities of this area and engage more critically with the issues.

*Care* – [Noun]: 'The provision of what is necessary for the health, welfare, maintenance, and protection of someone or something' (Oxford Dictionary online, Oxford, 2015).

*Care-giver* – [Noun] 'The person who provides the majority of care or guardianship, especially to a child or an infirm person' (Oxford Dictionary online, Oxford, 2015).

HCPC definition *Carer* – 'Anyone who looks after, or provides support to, a family member, partner or friend' (HCPC, 2015).

So what exactly is 'care'? Attempting to unpick the definitions above can bring with it more confusion. As a word, it was not until relatively recently that it began to be explored and debated as representing a phenomenon in its own right. Often seen as an identity or characteristic over which people have little control, the discrimination of a swathe of people brought care to the attention of theorists and academics in the latter part of the twentieth century (Larkin and Milne, 2014). The associated implications of dependency (of the person in receipt of care) and autonomy have been, and continue to be, critiqued by scholars and disability rights groups. This and the diversity of carers and that of the people whom they support is discussed in Chapter 2.

Leaving aside for the moment what could be crudely summed up as the disability rights vs carers' rights debate (Fine, 2014), if we then start to unpick terminology just by taking the *'provision of what is necessary for health, welfare, maintenance, and protection'* as a starting point, this covers a huge spectrum. There are many differences to consider, including geographical: for instance, for those living in the North of Scotland, the provision of heating is more necessary for health, welfare and maintenance than for those people living in Southern Spain, where electricity for air-conditioning may be seen as a necessity. Cultural differences, including expectations of filial responsibility also differ between a culture where there is greater emphasis on respect and family care for older people than is generally seen in the UK (Solé-Auró and Crimmins, 2014). Older age, as an example, is seen either as a time when one has achieved status and wisdom or as something undesirable, depending on the cultural expectations of the society in which it is perceived and experienced. The value that different cultures place on old age has associations with how caring for older adults is seen and practised, and these values can become internalised by both the recipient and the giver of care. Caring or care-giving is rarely delivered by one individual, given in one direction. It is not linear: for example, older adults may have more than one child who is providing care, a child more than one parent, and a spouse may have children and siblings to assist with care provision.

So, if we go back to the Oxford Dictionary definition, *'the provision of what is necessary...'* and this time examine the aspect of health, presumably this incorporates both emotional and physical health? If it is self-defined, then what I deem necessary for my own physical health – a long walk with my dog on a regular basis – and my emotional health – to relax and listen to music (preferably Bruce Springsteen) on a daily basis – may not be recognised as important by others. For those others, the ability to smoke cigarettes may be seen as necessary by them for their personal welfare and emotional health, and yet there is an inherent tension between this and the physical health implications that lead to this activity being condemned by others. Here again, this raises the question of who is actually responsible for deciding and/or recording 'what is necessary' and how does the subjective nature of the assessor make a difference?

Timing is also significant in any discussion regarding 'what is necessary'. To use the example of a parent-carer for a child with disabilities, the need for support to enable time to be spent with any other children in the family, perhaps in a practical way – taking them to school or attending parent nights – is likely to be limited by time, and is not likely to be seen as a 'need' in a practical sense for more than a few years. Likewise, the effect of some disabilities and some illnesses fluctuates. Provision of care for a partner who has multiple sclerosis, for example, is likely to be more intense at some times than at others, such is the nature of the physical effects of such a condition. Others may see the provision of 'what is necessary' as being more about those needs proposed by Maslow (1943). He described these as relating to physiological, safety, emotional (social), esteem and self-actualising needs.

Few would doubt the centrality of such basic needs as food and water, warmth and shelter. However, if you see my point above about the variability in these needs depending on one's individual circumstances, the question is posed about how and where these are obtained; are they provided for, and if so, by whom? Should they be provided for? Is there a distinction to be made between needs being met by someone 'giving' or of someone 'receiving'? Are they obtained or achieved? When we start to explore who, and what, is a priority for these 'basic needs' and how they are met,

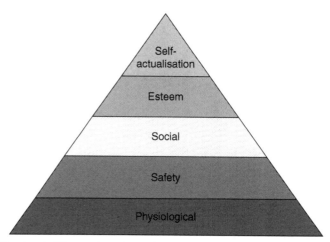

**Figure 1.1**  Maslow's Hierarchy of Needs

(provided, or funded) both contextually and globally this exploration becomes even more complex.

When needs have been identified – which may differ depending upon whether it is by self-identification/assessment, or by meeting some pre-determined criteria, which itself brings into question the subjectivity of any pre-determined category of need, how and by whom it is measured (Bradshaw, 1972) – the response to the needs of carers in any society is once again fraught with complexities.

So, the definitions are superficially complex, but lack sophistication. When searching the literature for others' definitions, the most common definition of carer and care-giving comes from the carers organisation, The Carers Trust: 'A carer is anyone who cares, unpaid, for a friend or family member who, due to illness, disability, a mental health problem or an addiction cannot cope without their support' (Carers Trust, 2017). Again, this is a very broad definition and makes no distinction between physical, emotional and financial caring. If, for example, I am worried about my 80-year-old grandmother and telephone her every day, she looks forward to the call and says it 'keeps her going'. To me, this is obviously 'caring' and yet it is quite different from an individual who may be providing 24-hours-a-day, hands-on physical care for their partner who has suffered a stroke and is unable to self-care, and who may require feeding, mobility and personal care. Clearly the individual circumstances and preferences, along with so many other variables, impacts upon the experience of carers and those in receipt of such differing forms of care. The internalisation of moral and social norms, access to resources, as well as the prevailing political ideology are just a few of the ways in which care and caring is identified, intensified and shaped by external and internal factors. If, as McNeil and Hunter (2014) suggest, the number of family carers reduces, this will be in direct contradiction to the demands placed on formal services, again at a time of cuts and budget reductions.

Vital elements in the Carers Trust definition above: the first is 'cares for' and the second 'cannot cope without their support' – both elements as we shall see in subsequent chapters are open to debate and discussion. For example, is 'cares for' taken to mean in a practical or an emotional sense? Might they be separated out? Likewise, on whose definition is the decision made that the family member or friend 'cannot cope without their support'?

The words care, caring and care-giving carry with them similar connotations, and yet there are differences, most notably between caring *for* and caring *about*. Care is itself an emotionally laden term. For example, I care *about* the current situation in Syria and the catastrophic impact the fighting has on children and young people, however do little in any practical sense about that. I care *for* my children in a practical and emotional sense, making sure their school uniform is clean, they have the train fare each morning, as well as whether they are happy, and have friends. I care *about* my students in that I want them to enjoy their programme of study, achieve a qualification, as well as learning and reflecting on that learning. I also care *for* my students in a practical sense, making sure they are offered an opportunity for a private conversation, and a coffee if they are distressed, and support them in their studies if life becomes problematic. In essence then it may appear that the difference between caring *for* and caring *about* are to do with practical elements, with caring *for* implying physical or emotional tending, and caring *about* a more abstract and temporal concept. An interesting question is whether one might exist without the other – can you care *for*, without caring *about* for example? As a family carer, one may go through the practical motions of caring *for*, without any thought of caring *about*. A wife who has experienced a lifetime of abuse from her husband who now has dementia may care *for* him in a practical sense, for example making sure he is fed and has clean clothes to wear, but does not in any sense care *about* him, and on more than one occasion may actually wish he would die. In another caring relationship, the geographical separation between a son and his father who has a terminal illness means caring *for* in a physical sense does not happen: however the son may be able to think of little else apart from his father's illness and may spend many hours each day searching for cures on the internet – is this caring *for* or caring *about*? I contend that both caring for and caring about take place along a continuum.

The emphasis on care, whether *for* or *about*, takes place along a continuum moving from no choice/moral duty on the left-hand side, to full choice and emotional wish to care on the right-hand side, and these may meet somewhere in the middle, reminding us that each caring situation is unique, and that care may be reciprocated.

No choice/moral duty→→→→→→→←←←←←←wish and choice to care

When you begin to explore the dynamics of care and care-giving – how it is understood by society, how it is arranged, managed and financed – you will see just what

**Table 1.1** Caring for and caring about

|  | **My children** | **Wife of man with dementia** | **Son of man with terminal illness** |
|---|---|---|---|
| Caring For | Yes | Yes | No |
| Caring About | Yes | No | Yes |

an abstract, political, social and ideological subject it is. Care giving and receiving is a fact of life and '...*not one of us can truly expect to look after ourselves through the whole course of our life without help from others.*' (Beresford, 2016, p 18). Care, therefore, is an essential part of human life and whether it is seen as a private or public concept, or a little of both, remains a moot point. Care (and care-giving) is both fascinating and replete with contradictions, dilemmas and debates, and a topic that requires a level of critical engagement in order to fully explore all its dimensions, and reveal others.

There is surely something ironic or paradoxical about writing a book purporting to inform, educate and offer a perspective on 'care' that is aimed at carers and the caring professions. You might imagine that anyone entering these professions does so out of altruism, out of a desire to help, to make other people's lives better and perhaps to empower.

In over ten years of interviewing prospective students for undergraduate and post-graduate social work study, I have found that one of the most common responses when questioned why they want to enter the profession is, '*Because I want to help people*'.

(*Note to potential students – you do need to expand upon that answer!)

For practitioners, a book to inform, educate and offer another perspective on the topic of care may appear to be self-evident. One would imagine that those in, or entering, such professions should have a clear understanding of the key issues and concepts relating to care-giving and will hold dear the values and skills needed to support a variety of people in a diverse range of situations.

This is not a 'How to...' book: the skills needed for working with, supporting and empowering carers should be part of every professional's training and education. Valuing people, treating people with dignity and respect, using open and honest communication and ensuring transparent actions, are the bedrock on which work within health and social care is (or should be) based.

This book is about trying to go deeper than those basic skills. In part it is about exploring the assumptions and prejudices that we all hold, and encouraging reflection and deeper exploration of one's own actions and those of others. I hope by reading this book you will question, discuss and reflect on the nature of caring in the twenty-first century, whether this applies to you from a professional or personal perspective, or both.

Being a practitioner in health and social care can offer a unique insight into what is, on many occasions, the 'hidden' world of care. I believe it is a privileged position. Care is, by and large, invisible; it takes place in the private sphere, generally behind closed doors. It can be messy, undignified, and extremely hard work, and yet it is a situation in which more and more of us are coming into contact, whether that be on a professional or private level (or both). Care is a great leveller, whether you are in receipt of it, provide it, or are in a relationship where both situations occur. The likelihood is at some point in our lives we will both provide and receive this slippery notion that is care. Surely, like death and taxes, if this is unavoidable it needs to be recognised as such, unpicked and articulated, and perhaps even celebrated?

Life is fragile, inestimable and unpredictable; unexpected events can and do occur. No one can predict exactly if and when they will be a carer, or if and when they will need care. We all have a limited time on this planet and need to begin to recognise and articulate that and, as suggested above, celebrate it for what it is, even though at times it may seem too short, too messy, and too complicated. This book will offer a discussion regarding the way society is organised, the (what I believe is a false) dichotomy between 'carer' and 'cared-for'. By so doing I hope it will introduce you to, or even expand your understanding of, discourses of care – including ethical debates – and will therefore, in some small way, help to inform and equip you with some of the underpinning knowledge and theories that provide the foundations for this most basic of acts – that of 'care'.

# Terminology

Language, the terms we use on a daily basis, and the meanings associated with these change rapidly (I still associate 'wicked' and 'sic' as negative things to be avoided). New definitions are included in the dictionary each year to reflect everyday vocabulary; for example, 'hangry' (bad tempered or angry as a result of hunger), 'mansplain' (the explanation of something by a man, typically to a woman, in a condescending or patronising manner), and 'me-time' (time spent relaxing on one's own) are all examples of words that appeared for the first time in January 2018 in the Oxford English Dictionary (see http://public.oed.com/the-oed-today/recent-updates-to-the-oed/january-2018-update/new-words-list-january-2018/).

In terms of this book it is important to set parameters and to explain what I mean by the different terms in use. For clarity, the following terms and their use are as follows:

> » 'People in receipt of care' or 'care-receiver' interchangeably. This is in preference to 'service-user', 'client' or 'patient', although I recognise neither

of these are universally accepted and that there may be alternative terms in use.

» I have used the term 'local authority' to refer to councils with social services responsibilities.

» The terms 'carer' and 'care-giver' are also used interchangeably to indicate a family member or friend who provides care to someone known to them, *without pay.*

» 'Health and social care practitioners' is, I recognise, a somewhat cumbersome term, therefore 'practitioner(s)' is used in this book to indicate anyone working with carers in a professional capacity. This includes students from a variety of disciplines, including social work, nursing, occupational and physiotherapy.

» By referring to the readership as 'practitioner(s)' as a shorthand, is in no way meant to imply that this book is solely for that audience as commonly perceived.

In addition, the text takes a broad view regarding care and caring as this would apply across all jurisdictions of the UK. However, where there are country-specific legislative/policy requirements, these are made explicit, as will be seen in Chapter 3.

Practitioners will often discuss the impact of knowledge, skills and values as these relate to caring and such considerations are often seen as a shorthand for notions of professionalism. It is therefore important to define how these terms refer to and impact on carers:

» Knowledge – Practitioners from a variety of health and social care specialisms working with and supporting carers need a certain degree of practical, technical and theoretical knowledge. This includes knowledge of legislation and its application, knowledge of benefits and the often complex financial arrangements that attend the caring role, and knowledge of services and support structures, all of which need to be located within the context of the condition or diagnosis of the person for whom care is provided, and effectively integrated (Hothersall, 2016).

» Skills – Working with carers, as working with those people in receipt of care, requires practical skills to make best use of the knowledge referred to above. Skills include communication: (Koprowska, 2014) actually listening to and *hearing* what is being said, and being able to interpret this meaningfully. For example, if I asked a carer about their typical day, and the response was '*Well I have good and bad days*', on a practical level it may be important to question this – a 'good day' might mean only being woken up twice in the night and having to change the bed once as opposed to several times, or it might mean that you were able to watch your favourite programme on television with only one interruption, whereas for people who are not caring this could be seen as a '(very?) bad day'. Clearly, therefore, skills of listening and picking up on nuances and subtleties are at the forefront of working with carers. Other skills include the ability to work across professional boundaries and disciplines in order to get the best possible support from a variety of professionals/service providers. The skill of being able to advocate effectively on behalf of carers should not be underestimated, as there can be real challenges here, particularly if a practitioner's assessment places what the organisation might feel are 'excessive' demands on its resources.

» Values – These act as a reference point for our decision-making and mediate both cognitive and emotional responses. It is important to appreciate that there may be instances where *professional* and *personal* values are challenged, and even compromised if these run counter to the values of the organisation or those of the carer or cared-for person (Akhtar, 2012; Martin, 2010). It is also important for you to maintain awareness as to the nature of the partnership between you, as the professional, and the carer. Do you afford them the same level of courtesy and respect for their views as you would another professional?

## Practical **task**

Take a moment to look at the professional standards and practice of the career you are in, or one in which you hope to join. As an example, for social work this is (currently) the Health Care Professions Council (HCPC, 2015), and for nurses, the Nursing and Midwifery Council (NMC, 2015). Read through the professional standards that entrants to these professions are expected to attain.

Do these conflict in any way with your own personal values?

Can you identify any instances where you think the requirements within the standards would likely conflict with those of an organisation?

As well as knowledge, skills and values, other attributes such as experience, wisdom, cultural understanding and a recognition of the importance of social and economic conditions (not least of these being access to resources) are essential when working with carers.

Looking again at basic definitions of the word 'care', consider for example the HCPC term *'look after'*. That too is fraught with contradictions and has different meanings applied to it by professionals and those involved in caring situations. Is it just about semantics though? Clearly it is difficult to narrow the focus of what is understood about care, although that does not, and should not, make it an invalid operation. Rather, through such processes, a consideration of these issues opens up broader debates regarding understanding and the use of terminology which, as we know, may be fluid and contextual. Regardless of the intricacies of the definition(s) applied to the action, we know, according to Carers UK and others (Dahlberg et al, 2007; Kudra et al, 2017) that 'care' is a situation that will touch the lives of millions of us at some point. Even if trying to capture the exactness and minutiae of the term is as impossible as plaiting water. The broader concepts and areas of understanding need to be discussed, reflected upon and broken down into component parts relevant to each unique situation. This text is designed to assist you in those processes.

# Structure of the book

## Chapter 2 Background to informal care

This chapter introduces you to the history of care-giving and it will consider what practitioners might learn from the past. Looking at the context for the carers movement, from the early action of one woman, to the politically active and nationally acknowledged organisations we see today, the chapter will trace the background to the ways that carers have emerged as a distinct social group in UK society in the twenty-first century.

Developing issues referred to in the introductory chapter, this chapter will set the scene for future discussions regarding the role of carers. The impact of legislation, social policy and the 'rhetoric' of community care on services will be considered in relation to the emergence of 'the carer' as will the impact of deinstitutionalisation and the move to 'care in the community'. Caring occurs within a relationship and this chapter will explore the reciprocity of care as well as looking at a range of ideas regarding the balance between the potentially competing needs of carers and those people in receipt of care. The chapter concludes with a discussion regarding the gendered imbalance of care-giving, and examines how caring is constructed as an identity as well as the significance or otherwise of this (Grimwood, 2016).

## Chapter 3 Law, policy, politics and people

Care has both an ethical and a political dimension (Tronto, 1993), and few would deny the moral, social and political significance of care-giving. This chapter will explore carers and law and policy, given that the current backdrop to care in the twenty-first century in the UK is set against a political ideology that emphasises independence, and values financial, material and career achievements. We know that carers are unlikely to have accrued savings of any significance and are unlikely to have access to private pensions. Carers are also more likely to live in low quality, privately rented accommodation. They are unlikely to have worked full-time and tend to be in low-paid, often temporary, employment. This chapter will draw on legislation and social policy to inform practice with carers. It is noteworthy that some of the problems carers experience may not necessarily be explicitly linked to their caring role. The implications of care-giving, set against a backdrop of austerity and financial prudence, will be introduced before being discussed in greater depth. The implications for practitioners will be highlighted.

## Chapter 4 Carers: caring and care-giving

Chapter 4 takes a practical focus, examining what it is that carers actually *do*. Through the use of case studies we will be looking at some of the practical activities undertaken by carers. This chapter offers opportunities to understand where and how support may be useful and asks questions like what are carers' workloads? What is the nature of the caring task? For many carers the experience of supporting and caring for a loved one, a family member or friend brings with it an enormous sense of satisfaction – of a job well done. What could be more important than seeing people you love and care about grow, thrive and survive, and know that in some (small?) part that is directly down to your involvement? For many other carers however care-giving brings about stress and physical, emotional and financial hardship alongside battles with professionals. This, and the adjustment to a change in the identity for many carers, is explored.

This chapter concludes by discussing matters relating to caring for children and babies, beyond that of the expected norm for parents, and a brief exploration of issues related to accessing short breaks and/or respite services, and what practitioners may learn from this.

## Chapter 5 Professionals and caring

This chapter draws on research that focuses on working with carers collaboratively in an interprofessional context. Who are the professionals and whether carers are professionals are just some of the areas considered in the chapter. Drawing on the work of Twigg and Atkin (1994) this chapter looks at the ways in which carers are viewed by professionals, and considers how they are seen; as a resource, a co-worker, a co-client, a professional or an expert? Are carers superfluous, and is their involvement viewed as tokenistic by professionals? Noting the feelings associated with 'imposter syndrome' by some carers (and practitioners) this chapter then turns its attention to matters of assessment of needs. The chapter concludes with an exploration of assessment, both carers' needs assessments and combined assessments under the Care Act (2014), and recognises the importance of multi-agency and collaborative work.

## Chapter 6 Research and practice

Continuing the debates begun in earlier chapters, this chapter looks at what research is and what it tells us about care and the effects of care-giving. Developing research-mindedness and intellectual curiosity are key skills for practitioners particularly in relation to care and care-giving (and receiving) scenarios in order to recognise the impact and experiences of such. The relevance of social media is also noted. The chapter will highlight the fact that care-giving is part of being human and the relational aspects of caring. The 'ethics of care' debate (Adhariani et al, 2017; Barnes, 2012) will be introduced and discussed.

As noted in previous chapters, carers are not a homogenous group and, as such, the emotional impact of caring will vary and be dependent upon a number of different factors. For many carers their situation is not seen as stressful or at all negative, and this chapter recognises some of the positive characteristics associated with caring. Concluding with a discussion of the importance of resilience both for practitioners and for carers, this chapter makes suggestions for further reading and inquiry.

## Chapter 7 Young carers, older parent-carers and carers of people with dementia

This chapter introduces you to the concept of 'care' as it relates specifically to three groups of carers: young carers, older parent-carers and carers of adults with dementia. While recognising that every caring situation is unique, there are however many similarities as well as specific characteristics that differentiate each 'group'. Using case study examples to highlight key points, this chapter also considers issues relating to students as carers and ways of supporting them to achieve their potential. This chapter emphasises the importance of clear and detailed recording by practitioners, and of agencies working together in order to enhance and support the work undertaken by family carers.

## Chapter 8 Reflections and conclusion

Safeguarding vulnerable people is everyone's business and this chapter will look at safeguarding inquiries, safeguarding adults boards and safeguarding adults reviews and offers a discussion of issues relating to post-caring, and matters of grief and loss.

The preceding chapters have been wide ranging, both conceptually and practically, in an attempt to furnish the reader with an outline of a multitude of issues relevant for carers, those in receipt of care, and practitioners alike. This concluding chapter summarises concepts, raised in earlier chapters to allow us to consider and discuss what the future may hold for carers, caring, and those in receipt of care.

Through an exploration of the 'metaphysics' of caring, a way through, or a gateway, into someone's world may be facilitated. Understanding caring is complex and nigh on impossible to appreciate fully. However, no matter how complex the situation is, and how many variables are involved, it is still a subject that needs to be pursued within the broader professional canon. Achieving a level of understanding regarding the lives of carers enhances what it is to be human, as well as enhancing practice and this final chapter attempts to synthesise some of the information and help support practitioners in the context of practice with carers.

In conclusion, care-giving and care-receiving are likely to touch us all personally at some point, and for those working in the health and social care professions, our professional involvement and engagement with care-giving will increase. As Kleinman (2012) so eloquently states:

*Care-giving is one of the foundational moral meanings and practices in human experience everywhere: it defines human value and resists crude reduction to counting and costing.*

(2012, p 1550)

For practitioners working with and supporting carers, developing their own insights and understanding leads to an increase in the building and developing of crucial relationships and may be the key to finding a gateway into that unique situation culminating in a deeper and more successful connection (Griffiths, 2017). I believe it is that connection and our possession of the capacity to empathise that separates us out as a species and offers hope for the future. As professionals, we are duty bound to do the best we can with what we have at our disposal. As human beings, we are morally bound to recognise the importance of caring and to accord it the status it deserves. As social workers, we must recognise the philosophical components of our work and try to understand the applications of such a perspective (Grimwood, 2016). This text will hopefully provide the basis for a more enlightened and engaged appreciation of one of the most significant roles and functions within society – caring.

# References

Adhariani, D, Sciulli, N and Clift, R (2017) Research Methodology. In *Financial Management and Corporate Governance from the Feminist Ethics of Care Perspective* (pp 81–117). Cham, Switzerland: Springer International Publishing.

Akhtar, F (2012) *Mastering Social Work Values and Ethics*. London: Jessica Kingsley Publishers.

Alzheimer's Association (2017) 2017 Alzheimer's disease facts and figures. *Alzheimer's & Dementia*, *13*(4): 325–73.

Barnes, M (2012) *Care in Everyday Life: An Ethic of Care in Practice*. Bristol: Policy Press.

Beresford, P (2016) *All Our Welfare: Towards Participatory Social Policy*. Bristol: Policy Press.

Bradshaw, J (1972) The concept of social need. *New Society* 30 March pp 640–3. London: Statesman and National Publishing Company.

Carers UK (2016) About Carers UK. www.carersuk.org/about-us [accessed 2 May 2018].

Carers Trust. About carers. https://carers.org/what-carer [accessed 26 March 2018].

Dahlberg, L, Demack, S and Bambra, C (2007) Age and gender of informal carers: a population-based study in the UK. *Health & Social Care in the Community*, *15*(5): 439–45.

de Boer, B, Hamers, J P H, Beerens, H C, Zwakhalen, S M G, Tan, F E S and Verbeek, H (2015) Living at the farm, innovative nursing home care for people with dementia – study protocol of an observational longitudinal study. *BMC Geriatrics*, *15*(1): 144.

Fine, M (2014) Nurturing longevity: sociological constructions of ageing, care and the body. *Health Sociology Review*, *23*(1): 33–42.

Franklin, B (2015) The end of formal adult social care. www.olderpeoplescouncil.org/docs/The_end_of_formal_social_care_1.pdf [accessed 26 March 2018].

Grimwood, T (2016) *Key Debates in Social Work and Philosophy*. London: Routledge.

Griffiths, M (2017) *The Challenge of Existential Social Work Practice*. New York: Springer.

HCPC Health & Care Professions Council (2015) Guidance on conduct and ethics for students. Information for students and education providers. www.hpc-uk.org/assets/documents/10002C16Guidanceonconduct andethicsforstudents.pdf [accessed 26 March 2018].

Hothersall, S J (2016) Epistemology and social work: integrating theory, research and practice through philosophical pragmatism. *Social Work and Social Sciences Review*, *18*(3): 33–67.

Hulme, C, Carmichael, F and Meads, D (2016) What about informal carers and families? In *Care at the End of Life* (pp 167–76). Cham, Switzerland: Adis.

Kudra, A, Lees, C and Morrell-Scott, N (2017) Measuring carer burden in informal carers of patients with long-term conditions. *British Journal of Community Nursing*, *22*(5): 230–36.

Kleinman, A (2012) Caregiving as moral experience. *The Lancet*, *380*(9853): 1550–51.

Koprowska, J (2014) *Communication and Interpersonal Skills in Social Work*. Thousand Oaks, CA: Sage.

Lamb, N (2014) Care Bill becomes Care Act 2014. www.gov.uk/government/speechesCare-bill-becomes-care-act-2014 [accessed 26 March 2018].

Larkin, M and Milne, A (2014) Carers and empowerment in the UK: a critical reflection. *Social Policy and Society*, *13*(1): 25–38.

Macnicol, J (2015) *Neoliberalising Old Age*. Cambridge: Cambridge University Press.

Martin, R (2010) *Social Work Assessment*. Thousand Oaks, CA: Sage.

Maslow, A H (1943) A theory of human motivation. *Psychological Review*, *50*(4): 370–96.

McNeil, C and Hunter, J (2014) *The Generation Strain: Collective Solutions to Care in an Ageing Society*. London: Institute for Public Policy Research.

Nursing and Midwifery Council (2015) *The Code: Professional Standards of Practice and Behaviour for Nurses and Midwives*. London: Nursing & Midwifery Council.

ONS (2013) Office for National Statistics 2011 Census analysis: unpaid care in England and Wales, 2011 and comparison with 2001. www.ons.gov.uk/ons/dcp171766_300039.pdf [accessed 26 March 2018].

OXFORD (2015) Oxford English Dictionary. www.oed.com

Robards, J, Vlachantoni, A, Evandrou, M and Falkingham, J (2015) Informal caring in England and Wales: stability and transition between 2001 and 2011. *Advances in Life Course Research, 24*: 21–33.

Smith, F, Grijseels, M S, Ryan, P and Tobiansky, R (2015) Assisting people with dementia with their medicines: experiences of family carers. *International Journal of Pharmacy Practice, 23*(1): 44–51.

Solé-Auró, A and Crimmins, E M (2014) Who cares? A comparison of informal and formal care provision in Spain, England and the USA. *Ageing & Society, 34*(3): 495–517.

Tronto, J C (1993) *Moral Boundaries: A Political Argument for an Ethic of Care*. London: Psychology Press.

Twigg, J and Atkin, K (1994) *Carers Perceived: Policy and Practice in Informal Care*. London: McGraw-Hill Education.

# Chapter 2 | Background to informal care

This chapter begins by looking at the history and evolution of care-giving and traces the background to the ways that carers and care-giving has emerged as a distinct social group and justified activity in society in the UK in the twenty-first century. Knowing more about the background to care-giving may assist practitioners to better understand the roles carers undertake and help to identify some of the relevant services for carers.

Focusing particularly on those carers organisations now known as 'Carers UK' and the 'Carers Trust', this chapter details some of the significant changes that affect the lives of carers in the UK today. Looking to the past may help in some way to predict the future. A discussion of community care and care in institutions is noted and the impact such ideology has on the lives of family carers is explored. Awareness of significant features from the past – for example, the move from institutional to community care – may help health and social care practitioners understand change, as echoes of the past inform the present and may shape how to work with, and understand some of the needs and issues faced by family carers today. The complexity of relationships involving a person with care and support needs and a carer is discussed with specific reference made to the existence of mutual or reciprocal care-giving. Although it seems the gap between the numbers of male and female carers appears to be narrowing, women still make up the majority of family carers and the gendered nature of caring is considered. Gender differences in the approach to, and expectation on, women as carers are also discussed in this chapter. The topics introduced in this chapter are complex, and invariably have been condensed; suggestions for further reading are made and throughout the chapter there are exercises and reflective points to support understanding and awareness.

How might carers be described? As family carers, as informal carers, as care-givers perhaps? If we take as a given that care in some form or another has existed as long as there have been people on the planet, and examples given below would suggest that this is the case, then questions need to be asked regarding the categorisation of the words mentioned above and the term 'carer'.

The notion of family and friends providing care is not a new phenomenon. According to bioarcheologists Tilley and Oxenham (2011), there is evidence that in Vietnam between 3700–4000 years ago an adult male appears to have survived for approximately ten years with severe disabilities which meant he would have been dependent on assistance from others for every aspect of daily life. Their research showed how he was paralysed from the waist down with, at best, very limited upper body mobility. This meant his condition would be difficult to manage successfully even with modern medical and technological innovations. And yet he survived. Testament to caring perhaps? Similarly, studying the remains of older Neanderthals who had disabilities, as noted by DNA analysis, there were indications of healing, leaving Tilley and Oxenham (2011) to deduce that the Neanderthals had achieved a level of societal development where individuals with disabilities were well cared for by members of their social group.

Literature and art also remind us of the prevalence of caring, symbolising and reflecting issues of caring. For example, in Dickens' *Little Dorrit* (1857), Amy, the younger of three children, spent her life caring for her father, and Jane Austen's Miss Bates who, as the unmarried woman with no income, was devoted to the care of her ailing mother.

A brief exploration of caring scenarios depicted in the Art world leads us to references to the tale known as 'Roman Charity' regarding Cimon and Pero, pictured on a first century fresco in Pompeii. The story goes that an old man, Cimon, was imprisoned for life without food; somehow, Pero, his daughter, gained access to his cell and in order that he survive, each night fed him her breast-milk. Cimon was later released from prison as an act of mercy owing to the fact his captors were so impressed by the caring act of his daughter. This image has been reproduced by artists throughout the centuries, including perhaps most notably, Rubens.

## Reflective **task**

Can you remember when you first became aware of the term 'carer' in relation to the definitions suggested in this book, or when you first realised that some people needed support in ways that perhaps you did/do not?

The reflective task above may be a tricky one for a lot of people. 'Care' can be a slippery term and to attempt to locate an 'epiphany' of when one first became aware of the word in its current form will, I suspect, be difficult. It seems to be a word that in many instances has been absorbed into common parlance, particularly for many of those in the health and social care professions. However, if care and care-giving as processes or actions have been an implicit part of some people's life-course over generations without the need for a specific 'categorisation', it is important to trace the origins of the word and to find what is behind the background to such definitions and the creation of such a category.

Like the word 'teenager' (attributed to Bill Haley and the Comets during a tour in the 1950s), and seldom applied or understood until the 1950s, the word 'carer' was little used until the 1980s and yet it is now becoming familiar in its usage. The following section will begin to explore where the development of the word 'carer' came from and the associations that are attached to it.

# Background to the carers movement

In the UK in 2018, there are many local and national organisations to support carers, either exclusively or in collaboration with organisations for people who may be in receipt of care. This has not always been the case and this section will focus on two of these, Carers UK and the Carers Trust, and will explore the background to their being established in the format we know of today.

The beginnings of public action that led to some awareness of what we now know as 'carers' in the UK, has been attributed to the Reverend Mary Webster (Carers UK, 2015). There is much to be learned from social history and Mary Webster's story is an interesting one. An unmarried woman without children, in 1954, she gave up her career in order to care for her parents, as was the societal expectation on unmarried daughters at this time. Faced with the prospect of poverty, having no income, and a likelihood of a stark future, this scenario may have gone unremarked, as it was for many other women in similar situations, were it not for a series of letters she wrote to the national press in 1963. Mary Webster, or Ruby Mary Webster (M.A.), to accord her full title, was born in 1923 and, unusually for women at the time, was educated at Oxford University, before eventually being inducted into the church in 1950 as one of the country's first female ministers. The scene was set for Mary to have a high-flying career, both academically and theologically. This came to an abrupt end when, in 1954, she found herself having to give up both her career and position in the ministry in order to provide care for her parents. The experience of isolation and lack of support that she felt for herself and recognised for others in her situation became the catalyst to her campaigning. Her father died in 1959 and it was towards the end of her mother's life in 1963 (note that is nine years after she gave up her career) that Mary, then aged 40, began campaigning in earnest. Articulate and knowledgeable, Mary was invited to give interviews to the press following letters she wrote to the *Guardian* newspaper (Carers UK, 2015) and further press involvement including radio appearances followed. Mary described her situation when caring for her parents as similar to that of being under 'house arrest' and this statement clearly struck a chord with others in similar circumstances around the country. Remember as well, this was the heyday for print newspapers as a major source of information; few people had telephones and the internet was still a long way off.

Parallels may be drawn between Mary's experiences of caring in the 1950s and 1960s and caring today. Indeed, for some carers in the twenty-first century, it would appear that little has changed. The feeling of being isolated and of being under 'house arrest' or 'entrapped' is one many carers still relate to today (Martin et al, 2006). It is now over 50 years since Mary Webster wrote her first letter to the *Guardian* newspaper.

As with many crusades or projects, timing is everything and it is important to recognise that the 1960s was an era of campaigning in many societies, and a time where the rights of others were beginning to be articulated and noticed, if not necessarily acted upon. Civil rights, women's rights, gay rights, and the rights of disabled people all began to take shape in some form or another. Although it is true to say that the impact of these didn't begin to appear until the 1970s (and beyond), the catalyst of much societal change in the UK began in the 1960s, which saw the start of the underpinnings of a 'social revolution' – for example, the liberalisation of social laws in relation to divorce and abortion. We might only speculate had Mary been born into a different time, what the outcome might have been.

By June 1963 Mary Webster and her supporters had lobbied Parliament. The formation of a group for women in similar situations to Mary, the National Council for the Single Woman and her Dependents (NCSWD), soon followed. Mary was in a key organisational role in the NCSWD as treasurer. As stated above, timing is everything. Not only were the social conditions right at that time – were Mary's mother still alive and Mary providing care – it is unlikely that her campaigning would have developed as it did, as on a practical and emotional level it may be assumed that she would have been unlikely to have had the time or energy to do so.

The NCSWD was an active group; they lobbied the treasury which eventually led to tax allowances and pension rights for women in similar circumstances to Mary and became the foundation of what we know of today as 'attendance allowance'.*

The NCSWD also campaigned for respite services and support for carers, including specific areas of support, such as bereavement counselling. It aimed to bring women with caring responsibilities together to try to address the isolation many experienced. Again, it is possible to see in these early campaigns echoes of requests for and services provided by the many carers' centres across the UK today. Although originally only single women as carers were recognised, following the campaigning of Mary Webster and her followers, the council broadened its remit and the NCSWD became the National Council for Carers and their Elderly Dependents (NCCED). However, this still excluded many carers, for example spouses and people caring for children. In 1981 this changed, with the founding of the Association of Carers. This was an organisation for all carers and was established by Judith Oliver, a carer for her disabled husband. Notably, this was the first organisation that was set up for both male and female carers, married and unmarried and of all ages. One of the key principles of the Association of Carers was that it was not defined by the diagnosis or categorisation of the person in receipt of care. This association was for *carers* in their own right, and aimed to link up carers as well as campaign for support and recognition.

In 1988 the Association of Carers joined with the National Council for Carers for Elderly Dependents, to form The Carers National Association. This association built on the earlier work of both organisations and continued to give carers a voice and some level of recognition, but there was little or nothing in the way of practical services or support other than some respite breaks for carers.

In 2001, following devolution, The Carers National Association was renamed 'Carers UK', establishing 'Carers Scotland', 'Carers Wales' and 'Carers Northern Ireland'.

The woman who had started it all, Mary Webster, despite her obvious indomitable spirit and tenacity, died at the early age of 46. However, her legacy is a national movement for carers and may be seen as testament to her hard work, articulation and challenge.

The Princess Royal Trust for Carers, set up on the initiative of Her Royal Highness the Princess Anne, in 1991 and like the Association of Carers was one of the early organisations to acknowledge that *all* carers require information and support as well as recognition of their individual needs. The Princess Royal Trust was instrumental in charity fundraising and attracting donations that were then used to establish Carers Centres. Initially funded for only three years (in part by the Princess Royal Trust and in part by statutory services), many of these centres for carers were able to respond to the needs of many carers in their locality, without carers having to travel for miles to receive advice and information. Many of these centres became independent charities and were (and still are) staffed in the majority by carers or former carers.

Seventeen years earlier in 1974, Crossroads Care, a local organisation for carers in Rugby, Warwickshire, was established, following a story line in the soap opera *Crossroads*, where a disabled man was cared for at home by his mother. *Crossroads*, the television soap, attracted millions of viewers for every episode and its portrayal of a caring scenario, involving an adult with a disability, however far removed that might have been from the caring experiences of many people, was at least a start. According to Carers Trust https://carers.org/about-us/brief-history-carers-trust, a viewer of the show, Noel Crane, who was also being cared for by a family member, contacted the programme to compliment them on their portrayal of such a scenario. ATV, the company who produced the programme invited Noel Crane to advise on disability issues in the programme and then donated £10,000 towards the development of a project to support carers in a practical way. This project, Crossroads Care, established in Warwickshire in 1974, expanded across the country culminating in over 200 centres offering advice and support to carers and their families.

In 2012 these two organisations, the Princess Royal Trust for Carers and Crossroads Care merged to become the Carers Trust, providing advice, support and information to hundreds of thousands of carers, and having specific programmes for young carers across the country. These projects include young carers and mental health issues (their own and those of the person for whom they care) as well as projects in school to raise awareness of young carers and help children identify if they are carers.

## Practical **task**

As you will have noted above, there are many carers centres throughout the UK.

Find out where the nearest carers centre is to where you study, live, or work.

What services do they offer for carers?

What are the opening hours? How might these and the services they offer benefit carers who may be, as Mary Webster said, 'under house arrest?'

How is your nearest carers centre funded?

In general, carers centres are a useful source of information, advice and support for carers in order to help them access the services they need. Carers centres in many parts of the UK carry out carers' needs assessments under the Care Act (2014) and are an important source of information gathering for both local and national government statistics (see Chapter 8 for some examples of initiatives developed at carers centres throughout the UK).

It is important for practitioners to recognise that not all carers may want to have contact with, or assistance from, carers centres for a variety of reasons. These may include not wanting to accept 'carer' as an identity (or as some may see, as a label), or perhaps viewing the support that carers centres offer as 'charity' or they may be reluctant to meet with others who they perceive manage their care-giving situations more competently.

## Personal **reflection**

How many of us have felt we lack the confidence to walk into a roomful of strangers and introduce ourselves at times? Now imagine that situation when you might be exhausted, feel as though you do not look your best, and are pressed for time. In my own role as a carer, the first time I plucked up courage to visit my local carers centre I couldn't immediately find a convenient parking space. This alone was enough to deter me for a few more weeks.

For many carers, having the courage to pick up a phone and speak to someone about their situation can be an enormous challenge, let alone finding time and motivation to go out and do so in person. Self-esteem and self-confidence become eroded the more isolated you become, and for carers this may be no different. Health and social care practitioners need to recognise this; simply providing information to a carer about their nearest centre may not be enough and I believe we have responsibilities as busy professionals not to make an assumption about this.

For example, in case notes I have read:

*I provided Mrs Smith with a leaflet giving information about the Carers Centre on ...(date).*

While of course people we are working with have autonomy to decide where, when and how to access services, a sensitive practitioner should be able to recognise that it is never as straightforward as merely providing information and then leaving it at that. There may be a myriad of reasons why this is not followed through by carers.

If you completed the task above asking you to locate your nearest carers centre, you may have found that carers centres generally offer services such as listening services, financial and welfare benefits advice, counselling, advocacy, support with referrals to health and social services as well as advice and guidance about 'respite' or short break services – clearly a really useful resource for many carers and may be a source of informal support and friendship as well. However, remember that the issues for many carers may be more about the confidence to seek out such services rather than the potential benefits of such. Family carers may have been encouraged to consider them-selves as such following completion of the 2001 Census – this was the first census to include questions on unpaid care (although the general household survey had included some relevant questions beforehand).

The Census 2001 (and again in 2011) asked the question: *'Do you look after, or give any help or support to, family members, friends or neighbours or others because of: long-term physical or mental ill health or disability or problems related to old age?'*

Options for answers were: No, Yes: 1–19 hours, Yes: 20–49 hours, Yes: 50+ hours (ONS, 2013). Results (for the UK) indicated that:

1–19 hours of unpaid care a week were provided by 4,060,706 people.

20–49 hours of unpaid care a week were provided by 897,374 people.

50 hours of unpaid care a week or more were provided by 1,548,377 people.

The provision of unpaid care is an indicator of the number of carers as well as people with care needs and is used to help inform the government and local authorities. Census information assists in planning and allocating resources, including social support and advice for carers and is a key indicator of the recognition of a group of people unacknowledged until relatively recently – family carers.

# History and development of organisations, policy and legislation relevant to carers

| History and development of organisations, policy and legislation relevant to carers |
|---|
| **1965** – Founding of the first Carers Organisation – National Council for the Single Woman and her Dependants (NCSWD). |
| **1967** – Dependent Relative Tax Allowance – the first legal right for carers. |
| **1976** – The introduction of Invalid Care Allowance. The first benefit for carers, but only for those who were unmarried. |
| **1981** – Founding of The Association of Carers, an organisation for all carers. |
| **1985** – Questions added to the General Household Survey (GHS). |
| **1986** – Disabled Persons Act (required LAs to *'have regard to the ability of that other person to continue to provide such care on a regular basis'*). The first time carers were mentioned in social care legislation. |
| **1990** – NHS and Community Care Act (carers receive recognition under that name). |
| **1995** – Carers (Recognition & Services) Act – provides for the assessment of the ability of carers to provide care, introducing the concept of carers' assessment. |
| **1997** – General Election – for the first time all 3 major parties' election manifestos included pledges for carers. |
| **1999** – First National Carers Strategy: *'Caring about Carers'*. |
| **2000** – Carers & Disabled Children Act (made provision about the assessment of carers' needs). |
| **2001** – Censuses – first to include question on unpaid care. |
| **2004** – Carers (Equal Opportunities) Act (extended the 2000 Act and placed a duty on local authorities to inform carers of their right to a Carers Assessment). |

| |
|---|
| **2006** – Work and Families Act (extended the right to request flexible working to carers in employment). |
| **2008** – Revised National Carers' Strategy *'Carers at the heart of 21ˢᵗ-century families and communities'.* |
| **2011** – Census – The questions about unpaid care remained the same, which makes comparisons easier to achieve. |
| **2014** – The Care Act – aims to put carers on an equal footing with those for whom care is provided. |
| **2014** – Policy paper Carers Strategy: actions for 2014 to 2016. |

# Community care and care in institutions

There has been a major shift in the provision of care over the last century and having looked at the inception of the carers' movement and organisations to support carers, attention will now be drawn to the ideology that is commonly known as 'community care' and the underpinning philosophy of this.

With its roots in the years of Margaret Thatcher and the Conservative party in the 1980s, culminating in a legislative implementation in the UK under the National Health Service and Community Care Act (NHSCCA) of 1990, Community Care can be seen as a formalised approach to the care of vulnerable people. Defined as long-term care for older people, people with disabilities or mental health issues, care is provided within the community rather than in hospitals or institutions. Community care was characterised by the closure of long-stay hospitals and heralded by two major pieces of policy and legislation:

> **1989** *Caring for People: Community Care in the Next Decade and Beyond* (Department of Health 1989). This White Paper set out the principles for a shift to community care, seen by many as rolling back State intervention in family life and reducing welfare dependency and culminated in:

> **1990** National Health Service and Community Care Act.

The ideal model of support for people in need of care became seen as the mixed economy of care: that is, a combination of care provided by the State, voluntary organisations, private sector agencies and family members. Underpinned by notions of economy, and financial restraint on behalf of the State, the emphasis on care provision was that it would be more appropriate to provide it outside of long-stay institutions and hospitals. Such promotion of independence for those people formerly 'detained' in such long-stay hospitals was seen by many as good practice and a reason to be applauded. However, the reforms to social care also ensured that more and more care would be delivered, not by paid and trained workers, but by family members and friends – those whom we now call carers (Carers Trust, 2015). This new direction in policy was seen by many as being instigated by economics and a wish to limit public spending. The policies and ideals underpinning community care have been criticised by feminists before, during and after its formal inception; for example, Janet Finch, in 1983, described it as 'care by the community', meaning care by the family, and care by the family meaning care by women (Finch, 1983). In 1998 the government aimed to take further action to reduce institutional care (Oliver et al, 2012), and continue to develop alternatives in the community through a number of measures, including amongst them greater emphasis on rehabilitation and more support for carers.

As suggested earlier in this chapter, the past can tell us so much about the present and the future, particularly when examining the reasons why people were placed in institutions originally. Incarceration in long-term hospitals can be traced back to the 1913 Mental Incapacity Act and before, which led to thousands of men, women and children being locked away for years, with the 'diagnosis' of being 'feeble-minded' or 'morally defective.' The 1913 Act made it possible to institutionalise women with illegitimate children who were receiving poor relief, similar to reports of people being placed into institutions for what we may see now as abuse they had suffered, or minor misdemeanours.

Decades of care in the long-term institutions and hospitals has long been seen as questionable at best, and oppressive and abusive at worst (Maxwell et al, 2006). A series of scandals in some of these institutions and long-stay hospitals, or 'mental asylums' as they were known at the time, led to the beginning of their demise by Enoch Powell as Minister of Health in 1961, when he advised that all long-stay hospitals should be closed within 15 years. The intention was that long-stay hospitals housing people with mental health issues and learning disabilities were to be replaced by the notion of 'Care in the Community'. Reasons behind the closures of such institutions are complex; as well as the rising costs, there was a recognition that the system was depriving people of their liberty. A series of scandals and major inquiries into conditions and practices at long-stay hospitals and television documentaries such as 'Silent Minority' produced in 1981 (British Film Institute, 1981) which highlighted the conditions experienced by some people with learning disabilities and mental health issues at two long-stay hospitals in the south of England, were indicative of changing attitudes towards the care of people with learning disabilities and mental health issues.

Over 50 years ago almost every large town or city in the UK had one, often very large, long-stay hospital for people with mental health issues or learning disabilities in the vicinity. Usually built outside of the towns, in rural areas, these prime development sites have long since been turned into residential (often) luxury homes.

## Practical **task**

The names of some of these long-stay 'asylums' have been associated with insults and stereotyping.

Find out where the nearest one to your home/place of work or study was and what it was called.

What reaction does the mention of the name bring about to people of a generation old enough to remember it?

In essence, it appears that society was recognising that care within such large-scale institutions, for many people for decades, was ideologically flawed and this, combined with a recognition of the importance of human rights and individual liberties for all (coupled with, as some may cynically say, an idea of potential financial gain for some), led to the gradual and almost total demise of large long-stay hospitals and institutions. This closure of the long-stay institutions and subsequent selling off of what was generally publicly owned land has been described by Cockburn (2012) as being one of the most radical changes to affect the British institutional landscape since the dissolution of the monasteries in the sixteenth century. Whether one agrees with the notion of institutionalised care in large-scale institutions or not – and there is a counter argument that says people who lived in institutions were protected from the outside world – the reality is that in the twenty-first century good quality of care is highly dependent on the availability and state of mind of care-givers and the quality of the care relationship.

As mentioned above, one of the factors behind the demise of institutionalised care was the increased awareness of the inappropriate levels of restraint and sedation used to maintain people in institutions in the numbers we have seen.

Such deprivations of liberty are at odds with current recommended practice; for example, the deprivation of liberty safeguards (DoLs) are an amendment to the Mental Capacity Act (2005), the safeguards that ensure that people who are looked after in care homes or hospitals are applied in a way that does not disproportionately restrict their freedom.

There is an irony in that one doesn't need to be in a long-term institution to have one's liberty denied; for example, if one fast-forwards to 2014, with the implications and awareness that the *P vs Cheshire West and Chester Council* and *P&Q vs Surrey County Council* (better known now as the *Cheshire West Case*) has brought about, it is possible to see that liberty may be denied.

## Reflective **task**

During an assessment regarding an older adult with dementia, the carer, who is his daughter, admits that occasionally she locks her father in the house while she goes to the shops and the cash point.

Do you think this is an issue?

What would you do with this information?

# Impact of care in the community on carers

Care in the community policies aimed to reduce institutional care, cut costs and emphasise individual and family responsibility. Therefore with the closure of long-term hospitals and institutions came the emphasis on care provision by agencies and families. As documented elsewhere in this book, there are examples that caring, both paid and unpaid, may be incredibly stressful, both physically and emotionally. High rates of sickness and absence, and a high turnover of paid care staff (Islam et al, 2017; Kovner et al, 2014) is a testament to this. There is research evidence pointing to the fact that mental health problems and suicide are elevated in health care professions and carers compared with the general population (Goldney, 2016).

This raises a number of worrying questions. Although this is a complex issue with many variables, if paid carers are reporting feelings of stress and fatigue, being troubled, 'burnt out' or distracted in their care provision – when they are presumably able to 'clock off' at the end of a shift, *and* are in receipt of financial recompense – they are unlikely be in a position to attend fully to the needs of people in their care.

Note: this is in no way supposed to undermine the work of paid carers. Research evidence notes that many staff are paid at a basic minimum wage, often feel overworked, stressed and may be overwhelmed at how little they can achieve in the time they have allocated to do so (Carr, 2014). The people they support are vulnerable, and may be living in situations of deprivation. That there is a disjuncture between the pay and conditions of employment of paid carers and the responsibility entrusted to that role, may be seen as an indictment of the esteem in which carers in general are held within society.

What then of the experiences of family carers? Research by Carers UK has found that 40 per cent of unpaid carers have not taken a break in over a year while, for 25 per cent of carers there had been no break in caring for five years (Carers UK, 2017).

Access to short breaks was one of the main factors listed by carers as something that could make a difference in their lives. For family carers, their own energy levels, mental state and focus on the role is likely to be compromised in a similar way to paid carers. Additionally, this needs to be multiplied and coupled with an emotional or relational aspect to the care provision.

To have a person you love more than anyone in the world shout and scream in your face from just a few inches away, threatening you with violence, even though you know their frail body may not be capable of performing such an act, while saying they don't know who you are – as may be the case for many spousal carers for people with dementia – must be heartbreaking. The enduring strain of this would make many paid carers resign from their posts, or at very least phone in sick with stress and anxiety perhaps. However, there are rarely such opportunities for family carers.

Few would question the legitimacy of communities caring for those less able to do so. It is seen as the mark of a civilised society which supports people when, and how, they need it.

For many, care in the community was predicated on the presumed existence of 'informal caring networks', generally relying on women's unpaid domestic labour (Finch and Groves, 1985). This situation harked back to the days of Mary Webster, with women as providers of family care being the expected and unquestioned norm. With the move towards care in the community came the unspoken assumption that there would be family carers ready, willing and available to provide care. As in the past, such assumptions on the availability of an expendable workforce of people's unpaid domestic labour, is generally thought to refer to women, and makes the expectation that women have the time, willingness, skills, knowledge and ability to provide care and, as such, would necessitate a withdrawal (partial or otherwise) from the labour market, with associated implications on income, savings, pension and future career prospects.

# Carers' rights versus disabled people's rights and the importance of reciprocity

If we take the premise of care in the community to mean care by women, what then of the situation of women who are themselves in need of support in order to maintain their daily lives? What then of women who have impairments or experience mental health difficulties and are in need themselves of care and support? What then of women who had been incarcerated in the former long-stay hospitals and long-stay institutions, often with very little evidence to support their being placed there in the first place?

Feminist research on care in the community has been critiqued for being one-dimensional and for failing to take account of the perspectives of disabled women (Keith, 1992; Morris, 1991). Focusing attention on the challenges associated with caring has served to portray women who have care needs associated with disabilities as being a burden, and both 'passive' and 'demanding' (Keith, 1992). Care and disability should not be seen as binary, viewing disabled women with care needs as victims, and in need of care, is neither helpful nor appropriate and blurs the debate about State versus individual responsibility. Feminist approaches to research and discussions regarding disability have been criticised by Morris (1993) who made the point that feminism has all but failed to adequately include the perspective of disabled women and, when it has done, this has not been helpful. The stereotypes attached to the labels of 'disabled woman' and of 'carer' may serve to polarise opinion and make what might usefully be seen as a life-course approach to reciprocity and mutuality unlikely. Whether termed 'care', 'personal assistance', 'help' or 'support', the likelihood of interdependency and co-operation between all, to meet needs, is one that is high. Care need not be seen as a barrier to independence, rather part of a continuum with give and take on both sides of the equation.

It may be asked does *receiving* care look and feel very different from *giving* care? There is not usually a clear demarcation between being a carer and being in receipt of care as both situations increase one's vulnerability and, thinking about the ethics of care debate, the emphasis needs to be on maintaining and strengthening the 'caring relationship' as opposed to giving more power to a 'carer'. We may also ask: Are autonomy or dependence polarised and are they characteristics to be valued in their own right? People with disabilities and those with care needs may have no choice about who delivers their care, and not everyone with care and support needs may want to employ a personal assistant, or conversely want to rely on family members. The rights of one group of people, ie those with caring responsibilities, should not be pitted against those who have care and support needs. What is needed is a more relational model (Barrett-Lennard, 2013) within which issues related to disability and those related to care, can be located and lead on to understanding of the different (and at times, similar) needs of both. The complex nature of both care *giving* and care *receiving* relationships needs to be acknowledged. Depicting people who need care as dependent, and those who provide care as autonomous, denies the recognition of difference, seen by Jenny Morris (2001) as a key part of our humanity. Caring is essential to our survival as a species, therefore it should come as no surprise that reciprocal caring exists and is prominent in some situations (Gant, 2017; Howson, 2016; Lingler et al, 2008).

The fact that 378,000 carers are registered as sick or disabled *themselves* (Carers UK, 2015) but still recognise themselves as carers is significant here. Reciprocal, or mutual care, is a fact of life, which is particularly apparent when considering the situation of carers of adults with learning disabilities, although I contend it is replicated to a greater or lesser degree in most caring relationships. Walker and Walker (1998) found that one of the most significant factors in older parent-carer families was the mutually dependent nature of the relationship that existed between the adult with a learning disability and their older parent. Heller et al (1997) carried out research concentrating on support provided by the son or daughter with a learning disability when co-resident with an older parent. Heller's results showed that the most frequent type of support provided was 'keeping company', followed by helping with chores, sharing mutually enjoyable activities, and providing emotional support for their parent. They also noted that a level of satisfaction was derived from this mutuality of care-giving. Such reciprocity took on a more significant role as the parent-carer became older. Interdependence in this example took many forms, not least practical and physical – for example, hanging out washing and emptying bins. Reciprocal care includes emotional support as well as practical and physical support; for example keeping the older parent company and providing companionship, may be key features of the mutually supportive relationship.

Reciprocal care and mutual dependency are acknowledged in the Care Act within the Whole-Family Approach (Care Act, 2014, Section 12).

*The intention of the whole-family approach is for local authorities to take a holistic view of the person's needs and to identify how the adult's needs for care and support impact on family members or others in their support networks.*

(DH, 2014b, paragraph 6.65, Care and Support Statutory Guidance, revised 2018)

There may in fact be issues with this, such as those highlighted by Clements (2015) who noted the potential for 'rounding down', ie overlooking the aims, goals and plans of individuals to those of the family as a whole, which may be less ambitious – it is a complex situation – and while there is a positive emphasis of seeing the family in its holistic sense, it is also important to balance the individual needs within this (for both the carer and the person in receipt of care). Practitioners may well be able, through utilising this approach, to make more efficient use of, for example, a combined personal budget of an older parent-carer and their adult son/daughter who has a learning disability and the freedom to do so should be seen as positive.

In addition to the physical, emotional and practical elements of reciprocal care, there may be an economic element. Financial *interdependence* is a feature of many reciprocal or mutual caring relationships. The various benefits people receive – for example, the personal independence payment made to an adult with a learning disability – may become an intrinsic part of the general household income and it may be impossible to separate this out.

Care needs to be seen as a relational activity, however within that relationship issues of respect, fairness and justice need to be promoted. People have specific needs that arise from giving and/or receiving care. Both situations are overlaid by multiple and often discriminatory factors. For example, carers from a Black or minority ethnic community face additional challenges (Greenwood et al, 2016). Although there are similarities across all carers irrespective of race, gender and age, the situation of Black and minority ethnic carers may be made worse by racism and ethnocentric attitudes within services (Merrell et al, 2005). Stereotypes abound about the high level of family caring amongst Black and minority ethnic carers in the UK (Willis, 2012), which may lead to further exclusion from services. We know there are issues of hidden carers, amongst all carers, however for some groups this is amplified. Studies show that Asian carers, especially Bangladeshi carers, are amongst the most neglected and invisible of all carers (Merrell et al, 2005), and there are institutional barriers, including religious, language and cultural, often coupled with a lack of awareness of appropriate services by those carers and by professionals. The UK's changing demographics, with an increase in the number of older people means that the number of carers from minority ethnic groups is also rising (Greenwood et al, 2015). Carers from minority ethnic groups may lack awareness of availability of services and may have concerns about the cultural or religious appropriateness of such services. Growing older may be accompanied by ageist attitudes alongside issues of discrimination and oppression from society at large. For carers from Black and minority ethnic communities these factors may be compounded by the vulnerability of giving and or receiving care and these additional disempowering factors need to be recognised, and acknowledged by practitioners.

The ongoing care of people who most need it, depends upon many factors, but none more important than ensuring that the care which is available is appropriate and also that it does not undermine both the rights of those individuals providing it, as well as those individuals in receipt of it.

# Gender differences in caring

There are gender differences in caring, in terms of men and women's contributions to care provision, to the intensity, the duration and the tasks involved. If we look at the way the carers movement began, it was based on the premise that (generally unmarried) women provided care. Its very title – the 'National Council for the Single Woman and her Dependents' – indicates that it was (and is still) seen very much as provision being in the domain of women. Of course, this represented UK societal perspectives and organisation at the time, although as with all things, it is important not to make generalisations. It was not until 1981 that the first carers organisation for all carers was formed; this was for all carers, not just unmarried women.

The gender distribution of care is uneven, with women representing the greater number of carers (Betts and Thompson, 2016). The 2011 Census showed that almost 58 per cent of unpaid carers are female (Carers UK, 2015). The percentage of carers who are female rises to 60 per cent for those who are caring for 50 hours or more a week and women make up 73 per cent of the people receiving Carer's Allowance for caring 35 hours or more a week (Carers UK, 2015).

Caring generally has been seen as a female occupation. It is seen as 'women's work' and, as such, is ignored in the 'male gaze' (Herring, 2007). *'Care work is an act that, for the most part, women do; it is a gendered activity'* (Meyer, 2002, p 6). Referring to caring as 'informal' further marginalises the people who carry out the tasks of care-providing and has an implication of choice. Research has linked being a woman and being married as key factors to being an informal carer (Arber and Ginn, 1995; Shaw and Dorling, 2004). The 2011 Census in England and Wales indicates that the peak age for provision of informal care is between 35 and 64 years (ONS, 2013).

So, being female, being married and being middle-aged all influence the likelihood of one becoming a carer. Therefore we can see that although Clements et al (2004, p 6) states: *'Carers are not a homogeneous bunch'*, the reality for many is that caring is and always has been a gendered occupation (Arber and Ginn, 1991; Carers UK, 2015; Chappell and Hollander, 2013; Dahlberg et al, 2007). For example, a consistent finding from the research on primary care-giving is that fathers are less likely to be care-providers than mothers. Daughters are historically more likely to provide care than sons. Evidence produced in the 2011 Census suggested that there are further differences, for example, men do much less actual direct caring and are less likely to be the main carer. Additionally, men provide care for fewer hours than women. The actual emotional approach towards caring by men and women may also differ, with males appearing to be more task-focused and more 'practical', as opposed to females who appear to be identified with 'emotional' tasks, although such polarisation has been critiqued (Carroll and Campbell, 2008). A notable difference in the approach to caring by women and men has been put forward by Taylor (2002). This perspective indicates a different approach between men and women when faced with stressful situations such as those brought about by caring. Women who have an approach that is characterised by 'tend and befriend' protect themselves and their offspring, or close others, promoting safety and aiming to reduce distress. Whereas men, for Taylor, have a different reaction to stress – they are more likely to have a 'fight or flight' or attack and flee, reaction to caring under stress. Generally female carers report stress and burden more than male carers (Chappell et al, 2015), and lower self-esteem (Kim et al, 2007), although this is an area which requires much more in-depth research, given the number of variables.

The gendered nature of family care-giving reinforces that which exists in the labour market for many women. Women are socialised into nurturing roles from an early age, and the gender disparities that exist in family care-giving – albeit recognising that there may be a small shift – is further evidence of this. An understanding of how women internalise ideas and norms regarding the notion of appropriate gender-role behaviour is needed.

In employment terms women tend to be in part-time, low-paid work and are more likely to be affected by punitive fiscal policies and cuts to welfare benefits (Rummery, 2016). Women's 'over' participation in the provision of family care, is reflected occupationally in roles such as nursing, leisure, teaching and social work, typically lower paid sectors. Despite the fact that more women than men work part-time, so earn less overall, even in full-time roles a pay gap of 9 per cent remains with women earning less than men in every occupation group (even those where women outnumber men) (ONS, 2017). Therefore to understand women as family carers it is important to take into account the gendered division of labour, as well as its reinforcement through social policy.

Caring as an activity is imbalanced, as it is undertaken by some of the most power-less people in society (Tronto, 1993) – that is, by young people and old people. Those with limited political and economic influence are more likely to be involved. For example, the census indicates that in 2011 there were 177,918 young people aged 5–17 involved in caring, which is an increase in England and Wales of almost 19 per cent since the 2001 Census. The gendered nature of caring is also evident here with 54 per cent of young carers being female.

## Gender balance and age

The number of hours of care provision increases as people age, and the gender balance does eventually begin to shift, being almost reversed in later life, when married men are more likely to be providing care (Del Bono et al, 2009) (although the approach, quality and intensity of such care is open to debate – see earlier point).

Put simply, as men age they tend to take on more caring tasks, as both spouses or as parents (Dahlberg et al, 2007), a fact that may be overlooked by health and social care providers. Research indicates husbands and wives, as carers, are taking on responsibilities that their spouses used to perform (Calasanti and Bowen, 2006) which presents several challenges, not least related to gender identity and the importance of maintaining a role. For some carers, the impact of austerity means that there may not be a choice between who in the family acts as a carer, the rise in unemployment and part-time zero hours contracts means that whoever in the family, unemployed or on such a contract, may be the only family member available to provide care, regardless if they are male or female, young or old. In data obtained from the 2011 Census it appeared that there was a small shift from the 2001 Census between male and female carers, including as suggested above, more male spouses providing care for their wives than before. It is noteworthy that where changes do appear to have occurred in the gender balance it is less straightforward than may be imagined and commentators, for example, Da Roit (2007) sees this as being less about the consequence of men's increased involvement per se, but more reflective of structural factors that exist in society. This, therefore, represents a class difference in that it is typically limited to middle and upper class males. This is clearly a complex area, and there is not room within this book to allow for an in-depth discussion of gender roles; however, what students and practitioners need to be aware of is the importance of not making assumptions about who is a carer (and conversely who is the person in receipt of care). Practitioners need to be mindful that there is always a likelihood of reciprocal or mutual care in any caring relationship.

This chapter has looked at the historical background to the carers movement, recognising there is much for practitioners to learn from the past. The importance of a relational approach to care giving and receiving is noted, and the likelihood of reciprocal or mutual care between both parties is discussed. The chapter concluded with an exploration of gender issues in relation to care-giving, we will now turn our attention to the formal acknowledgement of carers within law, policy and practice in Chapter 3.

## Taking it further

1. For an in-depth look at institutionalisation see Walmsley, J and Rolph, S (2001) The development of community care for people with learning difficulties, 1913 to 1946. *Critical Social Policy*, *21*(1): 59–80. This excellent paper discusses similarities and differences between care in institutions and care in the community and suggests amongst other points that they are on a continuum.

2. For further discussion regarding the reciprocal nature of care in relationships see Herring, J (2014) The disability critique of care. *Elder Law Review*, *8*: 1. This article discusses the need to promote care as a relational, and the requirement to break down divisions between 'carer' and 'cared-for.'

3. If you are interested in the debates to do with deprivation of liberty safeguards, including issues of 'best interests' you may wish to look at Chapter 4 of Golightley, M and Goemans, R (2017) *Social Work and Mental Health*. London: Learning Matters.

# Note

* Attendance Allowance: A benefit for people aged 65 and over, attendance allowance helps with the extra costs of long-term illness or disability, which can be either physical and/or mental. It can be paid regardless of one's income, savings or National Insurance contribution record and is a tax-free benefit. (Carers with care needs can also claim Attendance Allowance for themselves and this will not affect their Carer's Allowance.)

# References

Arber, S and Ginn, J (1991) *Gender and Later Life: A Sociological Analysis of Resources and Constraints*. London: Sage.

Arber, S and Ginn, J (1995) Gender differences in informal caring. *Health & Social Care in the Community*, 3(1): 19–31.

Austen, J (2003) *Emma*. 1816. Ed. RW Chapman, 4.

Barrett-Lennard, G (2013) *The Relationship Paradigm: Human Being Beyond Individualism*. Basingstoke: Palgrave Macmillan.

Beresford, P (2012) The theory and philosophy behind user involvement. In *Social Care, Service Users and User Involvement* (pp 21–36). London: Jessica Kingsley Publishers.

Betts, J and Thompson, J (2016) Carers: legislation, policy and practice. www.niassembly.gov.uk/globalassets/documents/raise/publications/2017–2022/2017/health/2417.pdf [accessed 28 March 2018].

British Film Institute (1981) *Silent Minority*. www.bfi.org.uk/films-tv-people/4ce2b69b6c084 [accessed 17 January 2017].

Calasanti, T and Bowen, M E (2006) Spousal caregiving and crossing gender boundaries: maintaining gendered identities. *Journal of Aging Studies*, *20*(3): 253–263.

Carers Trust (2015) Brief history of Carers Trust. https://carers.org/about-us/brief-history-carers-trust [accessed 28 March 2018].

Carers UK (2015) Facts about carers 2015. www.carersuk.org/for-professionals/policy/policy-library/facts-about-carers-2015 [accessed 28 March 2018].

Carers UK (2017) State of caring 2017. www.carersuk.org/for-professionals/policy/policy-library/state-of-caring-report-2017 [accessed 28 March 2018].

Carr, S (2014) *Pay, conditions and care quality in residential, nursing and domiciliary services*. Joseph Rowntree Foundation York.

Carroll, M and Campbell, L (2008) Who now reads Parsons and Bales? Casting a critical eye on the 'gendered styles of caregiving' literature. *Journal of Aging Studies*, *22*(1): 24–31.

Chappell, N L, Dujela, C and Smith, A (2015) Caregiver well-being: intersections of relationship and gender. *Research on Aging*, *37*(6): 623–45.

Chappell, N L and Hollander, M J (2013) *Aging in Canada*. Toronto, Canada: Oxford University Press.

Cheshire West and Chester Council vs P [2014] UKSC 19, [2014] MHLO 16.

Clements, L J, Thompson, P, Goodall, C, Gould, J, Mitchell, E, Palmer, C and Pickup, A (2004) *Community Care and the Law*. London: Legal Action Group.

Clements, L J (2015) updated 2017 www.lukeclements.co.uk/wp-content/uploads/2017/11/Care-Act-notes-updated-2017-08.pdf [accessed 28 March 2018].

Cockburn, P (26/11/12) www.independent.co.uk/life-style/health-and-families/health-news/the-demise-of-the-asylum-and-the-rise-of-care-in-the-community-8352927.html [accessed 28 March 2018].

Dahlberg, L, Demack, S and Bambra, C (2007) Age and gender of informal carers: a population-based study in the UK. *Health & Social Care in the Community*, *15*(5): 439–45.

Da Roit, B (2007) Changing intergenerational solidarities within families in a Mediterranean welfare state: elderly care in Italy. *Current Sociology*, *55*(2): 251–269.

Del Bono, E, Sala, E and Hancock, R (2009) Older carers in the UK: are there really gender differences? New analysis of the individual sample of anonymised records from the 2001 UK Census. *Health & Social Care in the Community*, *17*(3): 267–73.

Department of Health (2018) Care and support statutory guidance. www.gov.uk/government/publications/care-act-statutory-guidance/care-and-support-statutory-guidance [accessed 29 March 2018].

Dickens, C (1857) *Little Dorrit* (Vol. 1). London: Bradbury and Evans.

Finch, J and Groves, D (eds) (1983) *A Labour of Love: Women, Work, and Caring*. Abingdon: Routledge.

Finch, J and Groves, D (1985) Old girl, old boy: gender divisions in social work with the elderly. In *Women, the Family and Social Work* (pp 92–111). London: Tavistock.

Gant, V (2017) Understanding of the Care Act 2014 among carers of adults with learning disabilities. *Learning Disability Practice (2014+)*, *20*(3): 28.

Goldney, R D (2016) Suicide by health care professionals. *Medical Journal of Australia*, *205*(6): 257–58.

Golightley, M and Goemans, R (2017) *Social Work and Mental Health*. London: Learning Matters.

Greenwood, N, Habibi, R, Smith, R and Manthorpe, J (2015) Barriers to access and minority ethnic carers' satisfaction with social care services in the community: a systematic review of qualitative and quantitative literature. *Health & Social Care in the Community*, *23*(1): 64–78.

Greenwood, N, Holley, J, Ellmers, T, Mein, G and Cloud, G (2016) Qualitative focus group study investigating experiences of accessing and engaging with social care services: perspectives of carers from diverse ethnic groups caring for stroke survivors. *British Medical Journal Open*, *6*(1): e009498.

Heller, T, Miller, A B and Factor, A (1997) Adults with mental retardation as supports to their parents: effects on parental caregiving appraisal. *Mental Retardation*, *35*(5): 338–46.

Herring, J (2007) Where are the carers in healthcare law and ethics? *Legal Studies*, *27*(1): 51–73.

Herring, J (2014) The disability critique of care. *Elder Law Review*, 8: 1.

Howson, C A (2016) 'This is the child I know, this is the child I love': older parents of adult children with learning disabilities: perspectives on caregiving and quality of life (Doctoral dissertation, Brunel University London).

Islam, M S, Baker, C, Huxley, P, Russell, I T and Dennis, M S (2017) The nature, characteristics and associations of care home staff stress and wellbeing: a national survey. *BMC Nursing*, 16(1): 22.

Keith, L (1992) Who cares wins? Women, caring and disability. *Disability, Handicap & Society*, 7(2): 167–75.

Kim, Y, Baker, F and Spillers, R L (2007) Cancer caregivers' quality of life: effects of gender, relationship, and appraisal. *Journal of Pain and Symptom Management*, 34(3): 294–304.

Kovner, C T, Brewer, C S, Fatehi, F and Jun, J (2014) What does nurse turnover rate mean and what is the rate? *Policy, Politics, & Nursing Practice*, 15(3–4): 64–71.

Lingler, J H, Sherwood, P R, Crighton, M H, Song, M K and Happ, M B (2008) Conceptual challenges in the study of caregiver-care recipient relationships. *Nursing Research*, 57(5): 367–72.

Martin, Y, Gilbert, P, McEwan, K and Irons, C (2006) The relation of entrapment, shame and guilt to depression, in carers of people with dementia. *Aging and Mental Health*, 10(2): 101–6.

Maxwell, J, Belser, J W and David, D (2006) *A Health Handbook for Women with Disabilities*. Berkeley, CA: Hesperian.

Merrell, J, Kinsella, F, Murphy, F, Philpin, S and Ali, A (2005) Support needs of carers of dependent adults from a Bangladeshi community. *Journal of Advanced Nursing*, 51(6): 549–57.

Meyer, M H (ed) (2002) *Care Work: Gender, Labor, and the Welfare State*. Abingdon: Routledge.

Morris, J (1991) *Pride Against Prejudice: Transforming Attitudes to Disability: A Personal Politics of Disability*. London: The Women's Press Ltd.

Morris, J (1993) Community care or independent living? In *Independent Lives?* (pp 147–72). London: Palgrave.

Morris, J (2001) Impairment and disability: constructing an ethics of care that promotes human rights. *Hypatia*, 16(4): 1–16.

Oliver, M, Sapey, B and Thomas, P (2012) *Social Work with Disabled People*. Basingstoke: Palgrave Macmillan.

ONS (2013) Office for National Statistics 2011 Census analysis: Unpaid care in England and Wales, 2011 and comparison with 2001. www.ons.gov.uk/ons/dcp171766_300039.pdf [accessed 2 May 2018].

ONS (2017) How do the jobs men and women do affect the gender pay gap? https://visual.ons.gov.uk/how-do-the-jobs-men-and-women-do-affect-the-gender-pay-gap/ [accessed 28 March 2018].

Rummery, K (2016) Equalities: the impact of welfare reform and austerity by gender, disability and age. In *The Coalition Government and Social Policy: Restructuring the Welfare State* (pp 309–24). Bristol: Policy Press.

Shaw, M and Dorling, D (2004) Who cares in England and Wales? The positive care law: cross-sectional study. *British Journal of General Practice*, 54(509): 899–903.

Taylor, S E (2002) *The Tending Instinct: How Nurturing is Essential to Who We Are and How We Live*. London: Times Books.

Tilley, L and Oxenham, M F (2011) Survival against the odds: modeling the social implications of care provision to seriously disabled individuals. *International Journal of Paleopathology*, 1(1): 35–42.

Tronto, J C (1993) *Moral Boundaries: A Political Argument for an Ethic of Care*. London: Psychology Press.

Walker, C and Walker, A (1998) *Uncertain Futures: People with Learning Difficulties and their Ageing Family Carers*. Brighton: Pavilion Publishing.

Walmsley, J and Rolph, S (2001) The development of community care for people with learning difficulties 1913 to 1946. *Critical Social Policy*, 21(1): 59–80.

Willis, R (2012) Individualism, collectivism and ethnic identity: cultural assumptions in accounting for caregiving behaviour in Britain. *Journal of Cross-cultural Gerontology*, 27(3): 201–16.

This chapter will explore the broader legal, policy and socio-economic context and will consider the relevance and influence of these domains upon both the conception(s) and the practice(s) of care, carers and care-giving. We will consider the extent to which the socio-political economy influences the nation's health, wealth and well-being, examining the issues associated with the fact that the backdrop to care in the twenty-first century in the UK is set within a political ideology that emphasises independence, autonomy and individualism, and values financial and occupational 'success'. In order to achieve this and to provide a clearer sense of how, where and why carers, caring and care-giving are located within this broader frame of reference, it is necessary to first consider what law and social policy are and what they do. This chapter will there-fore consider the relevance of law and social policy and consider how this might be effectively utilised in practice to support carers in their roles as care-givers and how it might enhance notions of well-being.

# Law and policy

A simple definition and representation of the law and policy can be gleaned from the following extract from Hothersall (2010, pp 21–22) who reminds us that:

*The law can be defined as '(T)he body of rules, whether formally enacted or customary, which a particular state or community recognises as governing the actions of its subjects or members and which it may enforce by imposing penalties (SOED 2007). Its main practical purpose is quite simply to regulate and, in some cases, restrict certain kinds of behaviour within society. Using this definition and understanding of its purpose, we can see how the laws relevant to social work, social care and other forms of human service practice have their broad effect. In essence, the law (usually what we refer to as 'statute law') acts as a set of broad principles to be adopted in relation to particular aspects of life. Laws are [then] given practical effect by policy.*

From the perspective of the practitioner, understanding law and policy as these relate to practice is much like ensuring that you are aware of the rules of a game if you want to engage in it effectively. In order to do what you need to do effectively, you need to know what is permissible, practical and legal. A comprehensive understanding of the law and policy as it relates to family carers and those being cared for is obtained from a wide and varied corpus but, in essence, would necessarily include knowledge of the following statutes noted in the box below, as these relate to the appropriate jurisdictions of the UK (including the devolved parliaments of Scotland, Northern Ireland and Wales).

Significant legislation with relevance to family carers:

The Care Act 2014

The Health & Social Care Act 2012

The Mental Capacity Act 2005

The Mental Health Act 1983 (as amended 2007) (E, W, S & NI)

The Mental Health (Scotland) Act 1984

The Community Care & Health (Scotland) Act 2002

The Mental Health (Care & Treatment) (Scotland) Act 2003

The Mental Health (Scotland) Act 2015

Adults with Incapacity (Scotland) Act 2000

Adult Support & Protection (Scotland) Act 2007

The Carers (Scotland) Act 2016

The Mental Capacity Act (Northern Ireland) 2016

The Carers and Direct Payments Act (Northern Ireland) 2002

[All of the above statutes have a range of statutory guidance/codes of practice and other documentation attached to them – see the links below or go to: www.legislation.gov.uk]

For further information on law and policy relating to carers in the devolved areas of the UK, go to:

England: https://carers.org/article/policy-and-legislation

Scotland: www.gov.scot/Topics/Health/Support-Social-Care

Northern Ireland: www.assemblyresearchmatters.org/2017/06/07/supporting-carers-in-northern-ireland/

Wales: https://carers.org/legislation-affecting-carers-wales

# The welfare state

The history of social care and that relating to carers has been referred to in Chapter 2, but all of this sits broadly within the purview of what is commonly referred to as 'the welfare state' (Fraser, 2017; Rodger, 2000; Spicker, 2018). The range of law, policy and other measures designed to address social need are products of the ethos of 'collective social insurance', introduced by the report of the *Interdepartmental Committee on Social Insurance and Allied Service*, chaired by Sir William Beveridge, and its report, published in 1942, was responsible for the enactment of the following statutes, which heralded the emergence of the 'welfare state' we refer to today: The Education Act 1944 (The Butler Act), the Family Allowances Act 1945, the National Health Service Act 1946, the National Insurance Act 1946, the National Insurance (Industrial Injuries) Act 1946, the National Assistance Act 1948 and the Children Act 1948. Today's legal and policy landscape is much more complex, more sophisticated and more responsive, but all of it has evolved from these initial statutes.

However, while these developments certainly went a long way to improve the social conditions of many of the UK's citizens, things were not perfect, and as we have noted in other parts of this book, the position of women, and of those who were carers, was poorly represented. Having noted some of the impact on carers brought about by caring in the community and some of the details about gender and caring, attention will now be paid to the distinction between health and social care in the welfare state.

As founder of the NCSWD, Mary Webster's campaigning was timely and appropriate; she alerted politicians to the fact that the welfare state (Fraser, 1973) had in essence overlooked something significant in its inception (apart from a few exceptions, for example, some prescription charges). National Health services are free, whereas social care services are means-tested, which results in many people having to fund or make a contribution to social care themselves. The difference in funding also in some way means that the two main areas of welfare are viewed in different ways by society. In over 50 years since the inception of the welfare state as we know it today, the difference between the two main services remains with, in many cases, only a fine line to differentiate a 'health' need from a 'social' need. For example, if someone needs bathing to keep them clean and ultimately to prevent them developing pressure sores, and they are unable to bathe themselves, is this a health need or a social care need? Similarly, is administering medication for someone who is unable to do so themselves, for whatever reason, a health or a social care need?

According to the Association of Directors of Adult Social Services, ADASS (2014), the situation regarding what may be defined as a health care need and what may be defined as a social care need is complicated, and the (thin) dividing line between the care that local authorities should provide and the care that the NHS should provide is governed by complex statute and case laws. For carers, knowing this is a complex area may be of little comfort. If practical and emotional support and advice is needed by carers to enable them to carry out or continue in their role, it may seem of little consequence as to who organises and funds it. The debates and disagreements of different professionals, organisations and agencies, coupled with potential financial implications, may be seen as another example of additional stress and worry that carers could do without.

However, and at the risk of generalising (although such generalisations are perhaps less 'sweeping' than one might imagine), of significance here is the 'fact' that many carers are less likely to have participated in the labour market, or will have had their work-life interrupted by their caring responsibilities and as such, are similarly less likely to have accrued savings of any significance or have the benefit of an occupational/private pension. They are therefore less likely to achieve any real financial security or success often expected by society in today's neoliberal, individualistic climate.

It is also worth noting that carers are also more likely to live in low quality, privately rented accommodation, with associated costs such arrangements bring with them. Such arrangements may well have no direct connection to the caring role per se; instead, such arrangements may simply add more complexity to the situation once the implications of care-giving are set against a backdrop of austerity and fiscal prudence at governmental level (Betts and Thompson, 2016).

# Census data

The census is the largest survey that takes place in the UK every ten years. Having first began in England and Wales in 1801, developing statistics that help to paint a picture of the nation and how people live, the census provides a detailed snapshot of the population together with its characteristics, such as ethnicity and occupation and helps to underpin funding allocation to provide public services. Providing a periodic count of the population thus helps inform and plan for future levels of need or trends within society. Despite, as we saw in Chapter 2, the term 'carer' coming into being mainly in the 1980s, the first time that carers were specifically mentioned in the census was in 2001, making longitudinal discussions problematic. Although comparisons may be drawn between 2001 and 2011, it will take time for a more detailed longitudinal comparison to occur. There are limitations of census data – for example, it provides a 'snapshot' in time as opposed to a rolling census to capture ongoing information about the population. Homeless people or those with nomadic lifestyles are not included in the census, and illegal immigrants and other people who, for a multitude of reasons, may not be registered, are not accounted for. Similarly, completing the required data relies on a level of understanding and truthfulness. The 2011 Census data (ONS, 2013) shows there to be approximately 5.8 million people providing care in the UK, and this is likely to be an underestimation (Carers UK, 2015).

As indicated in earlier chapters, demographic changes mean that this number is likely to increase. The act of caring itself may be unlikely to be a major problem, given enough time and the right practical and emotional support; rather it is those situations and demands that run alongside it which need to be negotiated on a daily basis and threaten to derail it at any moment that are the issues for concern. As noted elsewhere, carers should not be seen as a homogenous group with a single set of needs. However, recognising the existence of carers and utilising appropriate policies and support does mitigate some of the impact that caring intensively over a long period of time brings about (Yeandle and Bucker, 2007). Policy attention that recognises the contribution made by carers to society as a whole is a starting point, for without recognition of such contribution, coupled with an appreciation of the impact of the health, financial, employment and social disadvantages experienced by carers, little will be done to improve, or support, people providing care.

# Political ideologies that impact on carers

Ideology plays a significant part in shaping how we perceive and interpret the (social) world. Hothersall (2010, pp 53–54) notes that:

*Ideology refers to a set of underpinning ideas and values that inform thought, language and subsequent action. In relation to social policy, such ideologies are indicative of the extent to which the state should have a role in organising, controlling and providing welfare to its citizens. Simplistically, discussions around ideology and its capacity to inform and influence welfare provision have tended to be represented by a left/right schism which has tended to become more apparent the more that the 'welfare state', typified by reference to the reforms of the Liberal government from 1905 to 1914 and the post-war Beveridge reforms, has been seen not to deliver on its stated aims of tackling the 'five giant ills of society', today perhaps exemplified by incontrovertible evidence of continued poverty and increasing and more diverse forms of inequality.*

(Wilkinson and Pickett, 2010)

We can see here the importance attached to understanding the nature of ideology and its influence in relation to how notions of caring, carers and care-giving are conceived and subsequently 'constructed' through the power of ideology. Heywood (2007) defines an ideology as:

*...a more or less coherent set of ideas that provides the basis for organised political action, whether this is intended to preserve, modify or overthrow the existing system of power. All ideologies there-fore...offer an account of the existing order, usually in the form of a 'world view' (and) advance a model of a desired future, a vision of the 'good society'... and explain how political change can and should be brought about...*

(Heywood, 2007, pp 11–12)

It is therefore important to take note of the power of 'isms': political ideologies reflect differing views on the role of the State. According to George and Wilding (1994), any major ideological perspective is likely to be *coherent, pervasive, extensive* and *intense*. It is argued by some that the dominant political ideology will soon be that of Western models of *liberal democracy* (Fukuyama, 1989), and liberalism, which is effectively the ideology of the industrialised West, and can be conceived as a *meta-ideology* in that it has the capacity to embrace a broad range of competing, and sometimes rival values and beliefs. So-called *social liberalism* looks more favourably upon State intervention in relation to welfare and other aspects of economic intervention.

If we then take 'ideology' in this instance as meaning a set of ideas and thoughts that form the basis for political and economic action, the following ideologies can be seen to have impacted on wider society, and have had a particular impact on care and carers.

# Neoliberalism

Neoliberalism may be defined as an ideology that has at its centre 'the market' (Witkin, 2017) and encapsulates the notion of a managerial drive towards an increase in the economy and competition. The focus on specialised provision and fragmented services impacts on the lives of the most vulnerable in society and can be seen as very evident in the (re)structuring of social work teams within local authorities – for example: local authorities now routinely commission out services that were once their sole responsibility; fostering and adoption services are a case in point. When one is talking about 'commissioned out', some may say that the organisation providing the lowest bid is seen more favourably and that such a move highlights neoliberalist (the market place) ideology in action. Often the organisations which are outsourced to, are those 'for profit' organisations, answerable to shareholders and a management committee with an overriding aim of making a profit – this may create a tension. Few would doubt the reduction of the role of the State within welfare, as this is highlighted by reducing or removing public services (for example over 350 Sure Start centres have closed since 2010, according to *The Guardian* 2 Feb 2017). This places greater responsibility on families, and ultimately on the caring role. This comes at a time when, as we have seen in Chapter 2, the number of people needing care, and the level, duration and intensity of those care needs has increased.

## Neoliberalism and care

Social welfare reform as a result of neoliberal ideologies has had an impact on ideas and thoughts about caring, both those internalised by carers and wider society and those ideas and notions seen as 'external'. The dominant discourse of neoliberalism has meant that the ordering of welfare services has been structured around a business model, one that seeks and highlights competition and individualism. One of the major consequences of neoliberalism is its impact on care for both those in receipt of care and for those providing it. There has been a rationalising and frag-mentation of services which has served to load even greater obligations on carers, and this has intensified in recent years (Carers UK, 2016). Personal responsibility is highlighted and promoted. Thus, it may be seen as an individual carer's responsi-bility to provide care and to undertake the safeguarding of the person in receipt of that care. The restructuring of welfare services along the lines of the market, with its emphasis on efficiency and effectiveness, appears to be in direct contradiction to the philosophical underpinnings of the welfare state. Small-scale community initiatives, developed at the level of a roots-up approach, which may be vital in building resist-ance and developing the sense of community are not powerful enough to challenge the neoliberal juggernaut that appears to have insidiously crept into society unchal-lenged. Economic changes to society which seem to be captured by the re-structuring of welfare services, for example, the emphasis on individualisation, on autonomy and on managerialism, are likely to impact severely on the individual carer in their own unique situation.

Only surface level issues are dealt with, for example short-term support with chal-lenging behaviour, or lack of available services geographically (Innes et al, 2012), and these issues may become decontextualised in the lives of carers and of the people for whom they care, thus increasing the social maginalisation experienced by so many carers who might be seen as being always on the periphery of society. It is not just carers and people in receipt of care who may be disadvantaged by the rise of neo-liberalism. Practitioners may also find themselves in invidious positions when levels of competition in relation to neoliberalist ideologies are introduced.

> ## Case example
>
> Ethel (87) a widow, looks after her daughter, Mary (66), who has a learning difficulty. Ethel has approached her local authority as she is finding it increasingly difficult to manage Mary's care, in particular her personal care.
>
> If you had to pick one profession or discipline, which do you think would be best placed to advise, assess and support Mary and Ethel?
>
> » Health Care?
>
> » Local Authority Older Adults Team?
>
> » Local Authority Adults with Learning Disability Team?
>
> Remember, all teams may be mindful of their budgets as well as the need to be seen to work together.

Having to compete for scarce resources creates rivalry and may only serve to alienate practitioners with the focus of their work moving from the well-being and supporting of carers and people in receipt of services, to a focus on satisfying the demands of the market.

## Egalitarianism/Collectivism

A counter to neoliberalism is a form of collectivism, which was one of the underlying principles of William Beveridge, the liberal economist whose 1942 report influenced the founding of the welfare state. Focusing on the needs of society over the wants of the individual the *Beveridge Report* was seen as paternalistic as opposed to authoritarian (Langan, 1998), and was referred to above. These 'competing' *ideologies* are nowadays seen as forming the basis of the inherent tensions and paradoxes experienced by all professionals and academics in the arena of social work and social care.

Changes in demography can also impact on support systems. For example, the growing longevity experienced in the UK also applies to adults with learning difficulties. This means that people with learning difficulties are now experiencing a similar life expectancy to the general population, and this has effects on other services. For example, palliative care services and end-of-life professionals may have a lack of expertise and knowledge in relation to learning difficulties, and those learning difficulty professionals may have little expertise or knowledge about palliative and end-of-life care. The family carer is significant in situations such as these as they may function as a bridge between two (or more) services providers, with associated issues that this may bring about.

---

**Case example**

Jackie (44) is a carer for her brother, Bobby (48), who has Down's syndrome and early onset dementia (N.B. people with Down's syndrome have an increased risk of developing Alzheimer's disease in middle age (Stanton and Coetzee, 2004).)

Bobby has lived with Jackie and her family since their mother died 7 years ago. He has had contact with social services and health departments since he was born, as he has a congenital heart defect.

Over the past few months, Bobby has been 'unwell' in a non-specific way. GP referrals have been made to various health professionals. However, Bobby – described by Jackie as outgoing and friendly – refused to get out of the car when they arrived at the hospital. When the GP visited him at home Bobby refused to get out of bed and put his head under the duvet when spoken to.

Jackie says she is 'at her wit's end'; she is worried about Bobby who is rapidly losing weight, he is barely sleeping and she wants to know what you are going to do about it?

---

# Legislation and social policy

As can be seen from the box above, there are numerous statutes and guidance relevant to carers and care-giving (see Law & Policy section above) and here we will discuss some of these in more detail.

The Care Act (2014), for the first time in the United Kingdom, amalgamated 'carers' into social care policy and set out carers' legal rights to carers' needs assessment. Local authorities have a responsibility to assess a carer's needs for support where the carer *appears* to have such needs. This is a development from previous legislation, namely the Carers (Recognition and Services) Act (1995) which stated that in order to receive an assessment of needs, carers should be providing 'substantial amounts of care on a regular basis'. Within this legislation, access to assessment for carers varied depending on a number of factors, not least geographical location and availability of workers to undertake such assessments, and subsequently on the amount of support offered. This legislation was seen by some as a starting point for the legal recognition of carers and the place of carers as 'skilled and as experts' in their own setting as well as introducing the concept of a carers assessment (Clements, 2017).

In order to obtain an assessment under the Care Act (2014) carers need to be over the age of 18. Legislation relating to those under the age of 18 is supported by the law relating to children; in particular the Children and Families Act which gives young carers similar rights to assessments as those over 18 have under the Care Act. (For an in-depth discussion of some of the issues relating to young carers please see Chapter 7.)

An assessment is a critical intervention since that is the point where key information is gathered. Any assessment under the Care Act (2014) should establish a carer's willingness to continue caring as well as considering what the impact is on the carer, and what the carer wants to achieve in their day-to-day life (as previously noted not an easy thing to articulate, for anyone, let alone a carer, who may be stressed and sleep-deprived).

When examining legislation to guide and shape practice with carers, of particular importance to practitioners is the indication of the 'Whole-Family Approach'. Section 12 of The Care Act (2014) specifies that the regulations must include what must be taken into account to ensure an assessment has regard to the needs of the family of that person. This approach goes some way to recognise the significance of the family unit as a whole, as opposed to seeing the carer and person in receipt of care independently.

Paragraph 6.65 of the Care and Support Statutory Guidance (revised in 2017) (Feldon, 2017) notes that the intention of the whole-family approach is for local authorities to take a holistic view of the person's needs and to identify how the adult's needs for care and support impact on family members or others in their support network.

The significance of any other family members for whom the carer has responsibilities is therefore recognised. If both the person in receipt of care and the carer agree, a combined assessment of their needs can be undertaken, although it is worth noting that in the case of a combined assessment, both parties still need a chance for a private conversation with the assessor.

Personalised approaches and individual budgets can provide opportunities for the pooling of resources to meet the needs of multiple people living within the family unit. An example taken from 2010, Foundation for People with Learning Disabilities, highlights how this needed to be addressed:

## Pizza story

A community nurse visiting an older family arrived early when just the mother was home. They sat and chatted while waiting for the daughter to arrive home from her day service. In the meantime, a home care worker arrived and chatted to both as she cooked tea for the mother – half of a big pizza. After her 20 minutes were up, the home care worker left and shortly after this the daughter arrived home. While they all chatted and had a cup of tea, another worker arrived at the home. This worker was from an agency and had come to support the daughter to cook her tea – the other half of the pizza!

The community nurse was shocked, but the family was bemused – they assumed that the workers who had organised the support for each person knew about the other person's support. The community nurse was able to report the matter to her manager, who alerted both older people's and learning disability services. As a result, the agency worker continued to visit the family and supported the daughter in preparing a meal for both herself and her mother (2010, p 13).

# Personalisation and individual budgets for carers

Personalisation is an international phenomenon (Larkin and Mitchell, 2016) that influences and shapes many different policy arenas, in many different countries. In the UK the move away from the power held solely by professionals towards a system whereby financial budgets are held by individuals to self-fund their assessed care needs is known as 'personalisation'. This is seen by many carers as a positive move towards independence, choice and control (Moran et al, 2011). However, critics of personalisation argue that it is a way of covering up increasing cutbacks in services (Ferguson and Lavalette, 2014). Additionally, personalisation may place many carers in a managerial role, on behalf of the cared-for person, with certain responsibilities for managing budgets, recruiting (and retaining staff), managing public funds and general administration.

## Case example

Gill (58) is the sole carer for her daughter, Laura (25), who was diagnosed with cerebral palsy at the age of three. (Cerebral palsy is a collection of motor disorders that affects muscle control, co-ordination and movement (Miller and Bachrach, 2017).) Laura also has a learning difficulty, severe epilepsy, and problems with both sleep and communication. She requires round-the-clock care and support.

Laura's care plan identified a set number of hours to meet the needs it has been agreed the local authority will meet.

Gill's assessment recognised that she needs a break from caring. However, it is Laura who will be the recipient of this service (a monthly overnight stay in a small residential provision) therefore it is incorporated into Laura's care plan and budget (as well as being noted in Gill's care plan).

Laura and Gill use a personal budget in the form of a direct payment to employ personal assistants to provide tailored care to meet Laura's individual needs. Laura loves music and visiting the cinema and enjoys these activities with her personal assistants.

Given the case study above, what do you think may be some of the positives of personalisation for:

a) Gill;

b) Laura.

What do you think may be some of the challenges for both women?

Broadly speaking, ideas around personalisation and individual budgets ostensibly link into notions of choice and control; there are however two competing forces at play here. We have, on the one hand, individualisation whereby autonomy and financial achievement are seen as desirable and valued characteristics. On the other hand, the focus is on a relational or familial approach which can be seen as being in direct opposition to the concept of individualisation with the emphasis on the collective, on the importance of reciprocal care-giving and highlighting the importance of relationships and family obligation. These two (mutually exclusive?) discourses can be seen as having their roots in late twentieth century economics where a neoliberal approach to welfare became subtly embedded into the psyche of society.

## Exercise

### Law, policy and practice: the never-ending media task...

This exercise is designed to develop your ability to identify and analyse material relating to law and policy from the media and other sources, to identify core themes/components and to weigh up competing elements in order to be able to collect, collate and present information with confidence.

1. First, identify an article/news item from a newspaper or other media source that relates to a legal/policy issue. This might be around carers and caring, but it might equally be about children, adults, mental health, education, housing, substance issues, criminal justice, etc. – all of which may have a bearing on the caring task and the people engaged with that. Make sure you cite the source correctly.

2. Summarise the information from the news item succinctly and accurately. What is the crux of the piece – what are its main points?

3. Identify the statute(s)/policy document/s that relate to the news item and look at the executive summary of these. Make a note of the main provisions within these. Use www.legislation.gov.uk for access to all statutes and statutory instruments. For access to policy documents, begin with: www.gov.uk/government/policies?keywords=&topics%5B %5D=national-health-service&departments%5B%5D=all&commit=Re fresh+ results

4. To what extent does the news item relate to particular elements of the law/policy document/s?

5. Are there any specific messages/challenges for social work practice arising from the article in terms of what it is saying about such law/ policy?

6. On your own, and over time, continue with this type of activity and extend it to include observations from within literature/fiction/films/other media. For example, Robert Tressell's classic novel, 'The Ragged Trousered Philanthropists' is regarded as one of the finest examples of working-class literature – see https://en.wikipedia.org/wiki/The_Ragged-Trousered_ Philanthropists. Try to go and see this: www.theguardian.com/film/ 2016/oct/23/i-daniel-blake-ken-loach-review-mark-kermode

# Carers and choice

Understanding the dynamics of choice involved in providing care and support to a family member or friend with care needs is a complex task. Choice and control over one's own situation may be seen as contested terms and of a multi-dimensional nature (Larkin and Mitchell, 2016). Would carers choose not to care? What would happen to the economy if that was to occur en masse? Carers UK estimates that carers save the UK economy £132 billion each year – more than the total cost of the NHS (a figure unlikely to appear on the side of buses!). Care-giving relationships are discussed elsewhere in this book in Chapter 7. However, for many, moral, social, political and financial forces often combine to remove the choice of whether to be a carer or not. Issues relating to race, class and gender, as well as economics all impact on the (sub) consciousness of carers. Care is seen as both innate and as being placed on people. Gendered expectations still mean that women are socialised to nurture and to care, in a similar way that spouses and civil partners are socialised to care for their husband or wife 'til death do us part'. For practitioners, an awareness of their own perspective on accepted social and cultural norms is relevant here.

Take a moment to consider the issues in the box below.

## Reflective **task**

Think about your own family situation:

Are you 'next of kin'?

> Who do you think might take responsibility, and who do you think *should* take responsibility for caring for you or your son/daughter/grandparent/partner/mother/father/sister or brother in an emergency?

What about long term?

> Think about your own employment or current programme of study; would you be able to continue with that full-time if you had additional caring responsibilities?

Can the State be left to market forces? For practitioners this clearly presents a dilemma. Obviously it is important to work closely with carers (and the person for whom they care), developing a relationship to ensure that no health and social care package relies on an inappropriate level of caring responsibilities. Additionally, it needs to be established that any care provided by friends or family members is sustainable or is unlikely to impact adversely on the independence, rights and health of the carer (ADASS, 2014). The definitions of 'inappropriate' and 'sustainable' are debatable and will surely depend on one's own value base, skills, knowledge, cultural and personal background. The discourse around care implies that family care is readily available and is always the first choice. This does not allow an exploration of whether the support to deliver this care by carers exists or that people (and I include those in receipt of care here) would see it as an optimal way of meeting care needs.

The smaller family size, lower rates of marriage and increase in longevity – all key features of family life in the UK in the twenty-first century – all have an impact on a likelihood of any realistic choice carers may have, to begin or continue in their role. With the demand soon to be greater than the supply of family care (McNeil and Hunter, 2014), the pressures on family carers are increasing. This is an unsustainable situation and highlights a dilemma faced by many societies globally, although the response to this situation varies from country to country. 80 per cent of care delivered in the European Union is provided by informal and family carers, the majority of whom are women (Betts and Thompson, 2016) and different initiatives are being applied to both recognise and support the contribution of carers across Europe. Examples of this include financial support, so-called 'cash for care schemes' (Da Roit and Le Bihan, 2011), pension credits, time off, paid or unpaid leave for those carers in employment (Betts and Thompson, 2016) and support services such as respite, training and counselling. Regardless of how it is approached the issue of care and care-giving is a global phenomenon when it comes to providing care for older people, and those who are ill or disabled (WHO, 2015).

## Carers choice as a positive entity

Having a sense of free choice in being a carer is strongly and positively associated with a carer's well-being (Al-Janabi et al, 2017). We know that the majority of family caring takes place in the home, by untrained and unqualified family members or friends, historically women, mothers and daughters. We also know that this is increasing; people are living longer, many with chronic and acute conditions that would not previously have been the case. The 'baby boom' generation born post-World War II are now of an age where they may be carers for their elderly parents, and for some, carers of children, hence the so-called 'sandwich carers'. Additionally, many will be in need of, if not in receipt of, care themselves (Moen, 2016). Coupled with this is that, in all European countries, the rapid increase in the oldest will undoubtedly present a major challenge. In particular, support for those with care needs which has so far been generally forthcoming from family care may well reach its limits (Lanzieri, 2011).

Therefore it can be seen that such inequalities in society that continue to be maintained are now becoming even more apparent with the demographic changes noted above. With the increase in numbers of older people there will be a concomitant increase in demand for unpaid family care for older relatives. This, coupled with the pressure on the pensions systems noted by Foster (2014), will be of particular detriment to carers; in particular, female carers. Pension entitlement is linked to earnings and labour-force participation, and given the likelihood of sporadic career histories, combined with the probability of having little or no savings many carers will be approaching an old age likely to be infused with austerity. Given the huge social and economic contribution made by carers to society (Hamilton and Thomson, 2017), this situation could be seen to be somewhat unfair and socially unjust.

Potential workers who are restricted by their responsibilities are limited in their choice of employment (Smith et al, 2008). Clearly more research is needed to identify and explore new patterns and new ways of supporting the work that family carers undertake. How, then, do such inequalities brought about by caring lead to inequalities in employment opportunities and in society more generally? As a career trajectory, few would imagine an element of caring beyond that of raising children to be a part of life and affecting one's future career options. This is the nub of it; we need to encompass a normative attitude towards caring and care-giving rather than seeing it as an intrusion, or as an inconvenience, and embrace it as part of the/our life-course and not be surprised if, and when, caring raises its head at various points along the way. To do this, both care-receiving and care-giving need to be seen as public issues to which there is a societal recognition and responsibility.

There is tremendous pressure on carers and on those in receipt of care to assume that they will give or receive (or both), care and that this is the preferred and only option.

What is needed by practitioners is a truly reflective 'unpicking' of their own practice base that informs their day-to-day work and an acknowledgement, however challenging, of the insidious way in which caring is organised and delivered according to neoliberal terms. As Tronto states:

*A world organised around care would be organised very differently ... we need now to stop being dazzled by the neoliberal forms of resilience and instead have the courage ourselves to return to a forestalled alternative future, one in which care truly matters.*

(Tronto, 2017, p 39)

# Carers and employment

Challenges exist for both employers and employees in relation to working life, job prospects and career development when taking account of caring responsibilities.

Literature and information relating to the importance of an awareness of the existence and needs of carers is on the increase. However, the main issues continue to be dealt with as 'private' ones, as opposed to 'public' ones. The hidden nature of caring discussed in Chapters 2 and 4, coupled with the lack of economic power or status that is held by many carers, may be seen as a reflection of the value placed upon their role by the State. The articulation of the political economy of care is evident in social and public policies (Yeandle et al, 2017). How such policies support carers into (or back into) employment is unclear. Working carers' ability to remain in employment may be under pressure due to societal and familial expectations. The tension that exists in combining work and care, and for employers being able to support carers to do so, requires flexibility and resources including financial enhancement, whether this is supported through insurance or welfare. What information and guidance that does exist for employers – see, for example ACAS (www.acas.org.uk/index.aspx?articleid=1362) – tends to be guidance only and lacks 'teeth'. So, although employees have a right to apply for flexible working and although many employers offer (or purport to offer) more flexible working arrangements for carers – for example, time off for emergencies, and the opportunity to request part-time or compressed working hours – this is, in the main, unpaid and may be reliant on approval by a series of managers. According to the Carers Trust (2016) there are 4.27 million carers of working age living in the UK, 57 per cent of whom are women.

For many, caring may come at a price. Issues discussed in greater depth in Chapters 4 and 7 note the poorer physical and emotional health experienced by many carers. Of those carers who are employed, the Carers Trust (2016) note that one in five carers actually give up their employment to care; however, it is not known whether this is due to ill health, stress, pressures of work, pressures of caring, or what would appear most likely, a combination of all of these factors.

For some of the 67 per cent of carers who are employed (Carers Trust, 2016), the workplace may even be seen as a solace or a place of respite.

## Personal **reflections**

On my first day returning to work following an (unpaid) break, one of the most gratifying events was when a colleague made me a hot drink, and later when another colleague asked me what I thought about a particular project. Small insignificant details to most people, but the contrast between home and work life was stark. I had a lunch-break and could, on the whole, work uninterrupted on a project. Additionally, at the end of the month I would be paid!

Few carers are able to afford to take unpaid leave, for financial reasons, and many are reluctant to do so, even if finances allowed it, due to the detriment (perhaps unarticulated) on their career advancement or their perception of them being less than a 'team player'. Research by Thomson et al (2008) indicates that people with caring responsibilities are less well remunerated when undertaking paid work. Additionally, Thomson et al draw similarities between motherhood and carers' 'pay penalties' (Thomson, cited in Hamilton and Thomson, 2017). The employment rate for carers is at 67 per cent although, as stated in Chapter 6, carers' employment tends to be on a part-time, or temporary basis, which has wider implications, that may impact over a lifetime.

Caring is a universal activity and an important part of family relationships, and yet the hidden and often unspoken nature of caring means many carers may be excluded and segregated from mainstream society. For people without caring responsibilities, or with funds to make this less of an issue, there may be a tendency to over-generalise this segregation and exclusion from their own experiences (Tronto, 2017). Does this mean that there is less likelihood of those in more powerful economic positions to be able to empathise and put themselves in the situation of others? If caring is universal, surely those in powerful positions are not immune from the effects and implications associated with it.

'We do not see things as they are, we see things as we are' – as Anaïs Nin so eloquently stated (www.goodreads.com/author/quotes/7190.Ana_s_Nin). One's own situation, background and experiences shape the way we view the world and our own place in it and it is difficult, if not impossible, to be truly objective and approach the situations of others in a rational way.

Most (reasonably functional) families are typified by greater or lesser degrees of inter-dependence. This (sometimes messy) entwining of people and their relationships can often mean that a temporary (or permanent) transition to providing care may be seen as a certainty, as opposed to an unexpected and temporary diversion. The duration and definition of care and care-giving is likely to differ at various points across the life-course. However, a 'whole family life-course approach' needs to be actively embraced and internalised above and beyond the autonomy and independence model noted earlier. For me, although this is an ideal, it is easy to be cynical and imagine how this approach may just be seen as 'pitting' one family member against another and a way of merely broadening out the meaning of autonomy and independence.

The difficulty with this is, of course, that the one 'named' person may become the scapegoat for everything. Families are complex and with often pre-assigned, and gendered roles. For example, the 'tongue-in-cheek' statement below provided by someone being assessed to identify potential ways of meeting their care needs, resembles many conversations and comments I have noted over the years in families where pre-assigned and gendered roles become internalised. Consider the following comments and think about how they may impact on the likelihood of one sibling being 'promoted' as a carer for their elderly mother who has considerable health and social care needs.

## Reflective **task**

When carrying out an assessment you ask a question to an adult with care and support needs about family, you are aware she has children, and support. You are given this response:

*Yes love, I've got two wonderful children... Let me tell you about them. Steph, she lives round the corner, has always been a nurturing person, even as a baby she played with dolls with such care, and has always said she wanted to be a nursery nurse. She's at work now – she's a real homebird – I know she worries about me all the time.*

and:

*....her brother James, well he is away just now, he has always been a free spirit. He took a gap year during his time at university, you know, and he even travelled round South America on his own. He loves travel and adventure, he has always been such a daredevil.*

The challenge for you as a practitioner is to reflect how you might be objective about these almost 'throw away' comments. Some personality traits or characteristics may be highlighted and recognised above others. For example, Steph (despite her afore-mentioned nurturing personality) may well have backpacked alone round California and bungee-jumped from Uluru (Ayers Rock), whereas James (the daredevil, and by association unreliable(?) off-spring) during his travels round South America, volunteered for 6 months to support older people in a homeless shelter and worked with street children in a sports programme.

Judgements are made in a split second. Remember – all of us, as individuals, have many layers of identity, some highlighted and noted about others by ourselves, our families and our friends and as a professional undertaking an assessment, it is important to recognise these for what they are – one person's opinion.

# Austerity and implications for practitioners

The privatisation of many public services, with its aim to lower prices and increase competition and profit margins, is not a model easily applied to welfare services. The most vulnerable groups of people in society – and in this I would include carers – may be denied or have limited access to, and awareness of, these services. Care and caring relationships are dynamic, contextual and geographical, and are likely to touch everyone's lives at some point. The overall profile for carers is one of low income, unemployment, lack of savings, lack of home ownership, of experiencing poor health and of reliance on welfare benefits.

Women and men are expected to perform and respond to different roles within society and are socialised in part to both expect and embrace that. We know that women, still in the twenty-first century, earn less than men. Additionally, as noted in the previous section, labour-based statistics indicate that women are more likely to work part-time, in temporary settings and in less secure roles. People on low incomes also tend to have greater health needs (Howard, 2001), and live in areas of high deprivation. Figures from the 2011 Census (ONS 2013) indicate that levels of unpaid care are higher in Wales than in England, and that there is a clear North/South divide with the highest percentage of care provision being in the North West, the North East and the West Midlands. Without the work of family carers, formal care systems throughout the UK would be unsustainable with some geographical areas particularly badly affected.

Few would deny the central role family carers play in delivering 'care in the community' as it was intended, however, with giving and receiving care: is it about not expecting everything from one person? One person may have that special quality at one time rather than in an ongoing situation. Practitioners need to consider this and question if a wider support network is needed. An African proverb states '*it takes a village to raise a child*' – meaning more people than just parents have a responsibility and an obligation to guide, shape and support a child through to adulthood. Therefore, why not consider, 'it takes a village to care' – basically meaning that it takes a communal effort to support those with care needs, thus care-giving should be seen as a shared responsibility, not just the concern of partners, siblings, parents or neighbours. Care is always contextual and no two circumstances are exactly the same, and yet perhaps all may be involved in giving and receiving care and support. While it is helpful for practitioners to have a named person, a contact to have that ultimate responsibility, by sharing the practical (and emotional) tasks associated with care and by recognising it as a natural part of life to be embraced, not feared, a more egalitarian society may emerge.

## Taking it further

1. If you are interested in the development and evolution of the 'welfare state' and social policy, then the following are excellent sources: Fraser, D (2017): *The Evolution of the British Welfare State* (5th Ed). Basingstoke. Palgrave Macmillan, and Spicker, P (2018): *An Introduction to Social Policy* available at http://spicker.uk/social-policy/.

2. For an account of the debates to do with the health and social care partnerships you may wish to look at Glasby, J, 2017. *Understanding Health and Social Care*. Bristol: Policy Press. Chapter 4 explores integrated care and the needs of, and how best to promote, inter-agency working, while Chapter 8 focuses on issues related to carers. Policy and practice dilemmas are considered throughout the book which analyses community health and social care and makes interesting use of case examples to highlight the points being made.

3. For an overview of NHS nursing and continuing health care it is worth reading a fact sheet produced in November 2017 by Age UK regarding NHS continuing health care and NHS-funded nursing care that details the stages and process involved in applying for such funding: www.ageuk.org. uk/globalassets/ageuk/documents/factsheets/fs20_nhs_continuing_ healthcare_and_nhs-funded_nursing_care_fcs.pdf

# References

ADASS (2014) Guide for health and social care practitioners. www.england.nhs.uk/wp-content/uploads/2015/04/guide-hlth-socl-care-practnrs.pdf [accessed 29 March 2018].

Al-Janabi, H, Carmichael, F and Oyebode, J (2017) Informal care: choice or constraint? *Scandinavian Journal of Caring Sciences, 32*(1): 157–67.

Betts, J and Thompson, J (2016) Carers: Legislation, Policy and Practice. www.niassembly.gov.uk/global assets/documents/raise/publications/2017–2022/2017/health/2417.pdf [accessed 29 March 2018].

Carers UK (2015) Facts about carers 2015. www.carersuk.org/for-professionals/policy/policy-library/facts-about-carers-2015 [accessed 29 March 2018].

Carers UK (2016) Carers Trust response to the Carers Srategy. https://carers.org/sites/files/carerstrust/carerstrustsubmissiontocarersstrategy_aug2016.pdf [accessed 29 March 2018].

Clements, L (2012) *Carers and Their Rights: The Law Relating to Carers*. Glasgow: Cargo Publishing.

Clements, L (2017) *The Care Act 2014 Overview*. www.lukeclements.co.uk/wp-content/uploads/2017/11/Care-Act-notes-updated-2017-08.pdf [accessed 29 March 2018].

Da Roit, B and Le Bihan, B (2011) Cash-for-care schemes and the changing role of elderly people's informal caregivers in France and Italy. In *Care Between Work and Welfare in European Societies* (pp 177–203). Basingstoke: Palgrave Macmillan.

Feldon, P (2017) *The Social Worker's Guide to the Care Act 2014*. St Albans: Critical Publishing.

Ferguson, I and Lavalette, M (eds) (2014) *Adult Social Care*. Bristol: Policy Press.

Foster, L (2014) Women's pensions in the European Union and the current economic crisis. *Policy & Politics, 42*(4): 565–80.

Foundation for People with Learning Disabilities (2010) *Supporting Mutual Caring: A booklet for workers in services who are supporting older families that include a person with learning disabilities*. Foundation for People with Learning Disabilities.

Fraser, D (1973) *The Evolution of the British Welfare State: A History of Social Policy since the Industrial Revolution*. Basingstoke: Palgrave Macmillan.

Fraser, D (2017) *The Evolution of the British Welfare State* (5th Ed). Basingstoke: Palgrave Macmillan.

Fukuyama, F (1989) The End of History. *National Interest*. Summer 1989.

George, V and Wilding, P (1994) *Welfare and Ideology*. London: Harvester Wheatsheaf.

Glasby, J (2017) *Understanding Health and Social Care*. Bristol: Policy Press.

Guardian (2017) More than 350 Sure Start children's centres have closed since 2010. www.theguardian.com/society/2017/feb/02/sure-start-centres-300-closed-since-2010 [accessed 29 March 2018].

Hamilton, M and Thomson, C (2017) Recognising unpaid care in private pension schemes. *Social Policy and Society, 16*(4): 517–34.

Heywood, A (2007) *Political Ideologies: An Introduction*. Basingstoke: Palgrave Macmillan.

Hothersall, S J and Bolger, J (eds) (2010) *Social Policy for Social Work, Social Care and the Caring Professions: Scottish Perspectives*. Abingdon: Routledge/Ashgate.

Howard, M (2001) *Paying the Price: Carers, Poverty and Social Exclusion*. London: Child Poverty Action Group, Carers UK.

Innes, A, Kelly, F and McCabe, L (eds) (2012) *Key Issues in Evolving Dementia Care: International Theory-based Policy and Practice*. London: Jessica Kingsley Publishers.

Langan, M (ed) (1998) *Welfare: Needs, Rights, and Risks* (Vol. 3). London: Routledge.

Lanzieri, G (2011) The greying of the baby boomers: a century-long view of ageing in European populations. *Statistics in Focus, 23*: 1–12.

Larkin, M, and Mitchell, W (2016) Carers, Choice and Personalisation: What do we know? *Social Policy and Society, 15*(2): 189–205.

McNeil, C and Hunter, J (2014) *The Generation Strain: Collective Solutions to Care in an Ageing Society*. London: Institute for Public Policy Research.

Miller, F and Bachrach, S J (2017) *Cerebral Palsy: A Complete Guide for Caregiving*. Baltimore, MD: JHU Press.

Moen, P (2016) *Encore Adulthood: Boomers on the edge of risk, renewal, and purpose*. New York: Oxford University Press.

Moran, N, Arksey, H, Glendinning, C, Jones, K, Netten, A and Rabiee, P (2011) Personalisation and carers: whose rights? Whose benefits? *British Journal of Social Work, 42*(3): 461–79.

ONS (2013) People, population and community. www.ons.gov.uk/peoplepopulationandcommunity [accessed 29 March 2018].

Rodger, J J (2000) *From a Welfare State to a Welfare Society: The Changing Context of Social Policy in a Postmodern Era*. Basingstoke: Palgrave Macmillan.

Smith, S, Le Grand, J and Propper, C (2008) *The Economics of Social Problems*. Basingstoke: Palgrave Macmillan.

Spicker, P (2018) *An introduction to Social Policy* available at www.spicker.uk/social-policy/ [accessed 29 March 2018].

Stanton, L R and Coetzee, R H (2004) Down's syndrome and dementia. *Advances in Psychiatric Treatment, 10*(1): 50–58.

Thomson, C, Hill, T, Griffiths, M and Bittman, M (2008) *Negotiating Care and Employment: Final Report for ARC Linkage Project*. Sydney, NSW: Social Research Policy Centre, UNSW.

Tronto, J (2017) There is an alternative: homines curans and the limits of neoliberalism. *International Journal of Care and Caring, 1*(1): 27–43.

WHO (World Health Organization) (2015) *World report on ageing and health*. Geneva: World Health Organization www.who.int [accessed 29 March 2018].

Wilkinson, R, and Pickett, K (2010) *The Spirit Level: Why Equality is Better for Everyone*. London: Penguin Random House.

Witkin, S (2017) *Transforming Social Work: Social Constructionist Reflections on Contemporary and Enduring Issues*. Basingstoke: Palgrave Macmillan.

Yeandle, S, Chou, Y-C, Fine, M, Larkin, M and Milne, A (2017) Care and caring: interdisciplinary perspectives on a societal issue of global significance. *International Journal of Care and Caring, 1*(1): 3–25.

Yeandle, S and Buckner, L (2007) Carers, employment and services: time for a new social contract? CES (Carers, Employment and Services) Report No 6. London: Carers UK.

# Chapter 4 | Carers: Caring and care-giving

This chapter explores some of the essential elements that practitioners need to consider when working with family carers. Through the use of a case study example, some of the day-to-day activities as well as the emotional and practical realities facing carers are illustrated and examined. By highlighting some of the practical activities undertaken by family carers, this chapter facilitates critical and careful consideration of how practitioners may start to understand where, and how, support may be useful. Care is a universal activity and an important component of many family relationships, however at times it may be a challenge and place family carers under immense pressure. This chapter goes on to discuss the stress that may be experienced by carers and highlights the importance of clear and accurate recording by practitioners involved in completing carers' needs assessments. Themes relating to parent-carers of babies and young children with complex needs are explored and the consequences of utilising short breaks or respite care from a carers perspective are noted. The chapter concludes with a discussion relating to the identity of carers and offers some suggestions for further reading.

Care needs arise from a range of circumstances, including physical or learning disabilities, chronic illness, mental health problems, alcohol or substance misuse. Anyone can be a carer; there is no differentiation for class, race, age, or sexual orientation and as such, the characteristics of carers are diverse. However, within this premise lies the possibility that there are certain features which make one more likely to become a carer at some point during one's life. These include gender (discussed in Chapter 2), age, race and cohabitation. Activities performed by carers are often based on ideas of love, duty and responsibility and are usually 'invisible', carried out, as it were, in private and behind closed doors.

## Case study: what do carers actually do?

Sylvia Twigger is a 58-year-old female who resigned from her full-time job as a retail manager to care for her husband, Rob. Rob, aged 60, has multiple sclerosis (MS – a lifelong condition which can affect the brain and/or spinal cord, causing a wide range of potential symptoms, including problems with vision, movement, sensation or balance). Rob's condition has progressively deteriorated over the last few years. He has limited mobility and uses a wheelchair when outdoors. He has difficulty with cognition, and struggles with co-ordination as well as the ability to control his bladder on occasions.

The couple, who have been married for almost 40 years have two children: Kim, who works as a teacher at a nearby primary school and Gareth, who lives in New Zealand. Additionally, Sylvia's 91-year-old widowed mother lives alone ten miles away in a small bungalow. There are concerns about her memory and general vulnerability. Sylvia is in daily telephone contact with her mother and visits her twice a week when Kim comes to sit with Rob.

Paid carers visit Rob twice a day. In the morning they help him to get up, wash and visit the toilet and in the evenings they reverse the process. Since his diagnosis, Rob has gradually gained weight, and is now classed by his GP as being 'morbidly obese'. Because the house has stairs that Rob cannot manage his bed is in the lounge. He watches lots of television and, as he has a hearing impairment, becomes annoyed if the volume is turned down. He refuses to watch anything with subtitles, or to wear headphones.

The case study above has provided you with some basic information relating to Sylvia and Rob. It mirrors some of the information that may be provided on a referral form. Without turning the page, begin to consider some of the practical tasks undertaken by Sylvia. When your list is complete, turn over and see how it compares.

Some of the practical tasks undertaken by Sylvia:

» shopping

» cooking

» cleaning

» laundry

» personal care

» budgeting and finance

» liaising with professionals

» managing medication

» keeping company

» being responsible for ...

As we can see from the case study of Rob and Sylvia there are many activities of 'daily living' which are undertaken by everyone; surely all of us need to attend to personal care, to shop, to clean, to cook? However, there are several differences that may be applied here, for example, time limitation: Rob understandably wants to maintain as much independence as possible. One element of this is that he insists on trying to dress himself and this takes a considerable length of time. Rob's co-ordination is poor and his balance unsteady. He relies on Sylvia to pass him each item of clothing, to stand next to him, and to frequently physically support him while he painstakingly attempts to dress himself. Sylvia recognises how important it is for Rob to do this, but secretly wishes that he would let her do it. By the time Rob is dressed over an hour has passed, and more than likely he has shouted at Sylvia in frustration, and they are both feeling exhausted and irritable.

Sleep deprivation is well known to parents of babies and young children. I am sure that many readers will remember that feeling of total exhaustion brought about by being woken by the insistent cry of a newborn, the experience of feeding a baby several times a night, then having to function the next day – a familiar scenario to many. What is less familiar is when this situation continues for years, or in some cases, decades. How to continue with the complexities each day brings about on just a few hours' sleep is a situation faced by many carers. While I am in no way infantilising the experiences of those people in receipt of care, there are some issues that are similar, for many. For example, using the case study of Rob and Sylvia above, we observe that Rob will not be left alone even when he goes out with Sylvia; the practicalities involved in supporting him with mobility means that any outings need to be carefully planned and that spontaneity rarely occurs. For Sylvia, learning how to dismantle Rob's wheelchair in order to fit it into the car was a challenge. Despite being a relatively new model, it is still heavy and cumbersome. This makes outings a less attractive option and increases the likelihood of isolation and boredom. Sylvia has never enjoyed driving and until his illness progressed, whenever they went out in the car together, Rob was always the driver. Because of Rob's weight gain, Sylvia has difficulty pushing the wheelchair, and Rob is unwilling to get a motorised version.

Other differences in the tasks of daily living between carers and non-carers for example, can be that: often carers are solely responsible for performing those tasks for themselves (and for others) on a tight budget. As a very basic example, there is no spare cash for takeaways if they are unable to face cooking again. In the case study above, as with so many caring situations, mealtimes often present a conundrum. Sylvia has to cater for, and feed, herself and Rob. Taking this as a given, the actuality of this innocuous act is far from straightforward: first, Rob does not like being left on his own, so this necessitates arranging for a neighbour to sit with him while Sylvia shops. Sylvia is a proud woman and does not like to ask her neighbour for help, but she steels herself to do so once a fortnight. She relies on going to the (more expensive) corner shop in between times during the 30 minutes when the paid carers are with her husband in the morning. She tried online shopping once but found it confusing and stressful as the computer is old and internet access fluctuates. Before he developed MS Rob enjoyed cooking, especially making curries. The couple miss those days and find the current arrangement difficult to accept. (Remember, feelings of grief and loss do not follow purely bereavement; sometimes it is the loss of smaller day-to-day activities that bring about the deepest sense of sorrow.) Rob will frequently make suggestions for complex meals; however, Sylvia sometimes has difficulties both in finding the correct ingredients and in the time that it takes to prepare the dishes.

When the food has been purchased and brought home, Sylvia then has to cook it and make sure that it is something that will please Rob. He is frustrated at being unable to do this himself and describes himself as quite a fussy eater and likes things 'just so'. Sylvia will ensure that the food is at an appropriate temperature, and if Rob's co-ordination is poor, she will feed him. Additionally, because of the nature of his disability Rob eats slowly, which means Sylvia's own meal becomes cold, as does Rob's, during the time it takes him to eat. After eating, Sylvia has to clear the dishes away and tidy the kitchen.

Rob needs her to assist him to use the toilet and on occasions he loses control of his bladder and bowels, which necessitates a strip wash and a change of clothes. Additionally, on occasions, the chair Rob uses has been soiled and the cushion needs cleaning. Yesterday's laundry is still waiting to be dealt with. By the time this is sorted and the kitchen organised Sylvia is ready to sit down; however, it is time for Rob's medication, which he will only take with a cup of tea, and on occasions he needs Sylvia to steady the cup for him.

The above is just one element of day-to-day life and yet it is possible to see issues that resonate with the other areas listed above. There are fluctuations between days in terms of what it is that Sylvia has to do on a practical level. How might you, as a practitioner, tease out what it is that is happening here?

Take a moment to consider the other daily tasks listed above and what you think these issues might be.

The main areas of work and daily activity that carers 'do' is less easy to articulate. In order to qualify for Carer's Allowance one needs to be providing care for at least 35 hours a week. Quantifying this is relatively easy, although time consuming; for example, personal care may take three hours a day, emotional support two hours a day, etc. What is less easy to quantify are the overarching feelings of responsibility and the stress that may be associated with caring.

# Carer stress

It is well reported that carers experience stress at a higher level than those without caring responsibilities (Martin et al, 2006; Shah et al, 2010; Williams and Robinson, 2001). One such stressor that may be seen replicated in the case study above is that discussed by Pearlin et al in 1990 as being 'relational deprivation' or the 'deprivation of intimate exchange', which includes losing the closeness of the relationship.

*The sheer dramatic and involuntary transformation of a cherished relationship is itself a major source of stress.*

(Pearlin et al, 1990, p 584)

Although here discussing situations involving people with dementia, it is possible to extrapolate from this early work, themes that will resonate for carers of people with other diagnoses and conditions today. It is important to note that carer stress can obviously have a multitude of causes, not necessarily to do with the cared-for person.

Frustrations caused by support services and organisations not functioning as promised results in carers feeling let down and obstructed. Research by Williams and Robinson (2000) found that many carers reported that their relationships with professional services were more stressful than years of providing care for their son or daughter with a learning difficulty. In a similar vein, research by Todd and Jones (2003) highlighted the problematic dealings with professionals experienced by mothers of children with learning difficulties. The mothers in their study felt that any meetings regarding their child with learning difficulties were based on conflict and that their abilities as mothers were being constantly analysed. Williams and Robinson's (2000) research noted how carers of adults with learning difficulties describe their relationship with such services using the language of war. Carers spoke about 'fighting' on behalf of their cared-for person, and 'battling' to receive services. Another issue arises due to a lack of consistent communication between different professionals. One of the main frustrations experienced by carers is succinctly recorded by Mencap as (2006, p 3): *'It's not caused by caring – it is caused by caring without the right help'* – an example of this being the issue of dealing with professionals who do not appear to communicate with each other, and who rarely read their own organisation's case notes.

As noted above, the fact that carers experience higher levels of stress than the general population is well documented. Stress is not necessarily a bad thing; it can be seen as a warning, or can inspire one to move forward or change one's situation or lifestyle. Likewise, altruism, by focusing on the needs of others, has a positive effect on one's own well-being. The issues arise when there is no choice or control, and when supporting others comes at a detrimental price to one's own physical and emotional health (remember the adage 'put on your own life jacket before assisting others to do so'?). The complexities of caring within a family environment mean that the causes of stress fluctuate and may be difficult for carers to recognise and articulate. Studies indicate that the characteristics of the person in receipt of care are seen as significant in determining carer stress. A high incidence of behavioural difficulties such as aggression, self-injury, destructiveness and non-compliance is seen as more challenging than disability type (Roper et al, 2014). However, poor physical health and high physical dependency all contribute to greater stress levels experienced by carers (Floyd and Gallagher, 1997; Hayden and Goldman, 1996). As the population ages, more older people are likely to require support to meet their health and social care needs, and, this appears to be a situation that will increase. For practitioners the key skills of a good assessment, whether undertaken for health or social care purposes, are often those involved in picking up on nuances and subtleties, and the language used. Likewise, the same questions asked in the presence of the cared-for person are unlikely to produce the same response if asked when the carer is on their own. Recording facts and details are important: comments such as 'Rob has disturbed sleep' may mean something to the practitioner who records that, however for the next person working with the family it may have a completely different interpretation. 'Disturbed sleep' may be due to external noise, for example, fireworks at a New Year's Eve party next door, or a car alarm going off incessantly, or it may be due to severe pain or anxiety brought about by the nature of a health condition. This basic example highlights the importance of those health and/or social care workers who are carrying out an assessment to use factual information insofar as it is available. Therefore, 'Rob said he wakes up on average three times a night due to pain in his legs. When this happens he calls Sylvia to massage them, it usually takes 15 minutes to ease. As he is awake, Rob likes a warm drink to help him settle, and he may need to use the toilet' and the week prior to this report being written, Sylvia said that Rob had woken every night, each night they were both awake for two or three intervals of at least 45 minutes. Remember as basic as it sounds whoever is carrying out the assessment needs to include relevant dates – 'last week' will mean little to colleagues in six months time!

Combined assessments under the Care Act (2014) are possible if both parties agree, but they are not without problems and it would take a skilled and experienced practitioner to separate out the needs and to ensure that both parties are at the centre of the assessment process. Whose voice is heard and is loudest? Understanding the dynamics of care, interactions and dependencies between individuals, is invariably complex. Practitioners need to rely on their professional judgement to begin to analyse the information they have obtained in order make a decision about a situation. Carers' needs assessments are discussed in greater depth in the following chapter, however, it is worth noting at this juncture that the purpose of a carer's needs assessment under the Care Act (2014), is to establish whether (Section 10):

> » The carer is able and likely to continue to be able to provide care for the adult needing care.
>
> » The carer is willing and likely to continue to be willing (crystal ball time perhaps?) to provide care.
>
> » What the impact of the carer's needs for support is on their own well-being.
>
> » The outcomes the carer wants to achieve and if the provision of support could contribute to the achievement of those outcomes.

In short they must include the carer's need for support, the sustainability of the caring role and the outcomes that the carer wants to achieve in their daily life.

This is fairly amorphous; which of us, if asked, would be able to articulate the outcomes that we want to achieve in our daily life? There is an issue here for self-assessments, particularly those with pre-set boxes.

## Practical **task**

Without any preparation, 'off the top of your head', make a note of five outcomes you want to achieve in your daily life. Note how long it takes you to come up with the list.

Ask a friend or colleague to do the same and then compare them and see if, and how, they differ. Then set a reminder on your phone to re-visit your list in six months time. See what, and if any, changes there are.

Without an experienced professional to ask the 'right' sort of questions, to prompt and remind people to pick up on and explore subtle nuances and inferences, a distorted picture may be produced of what it actually is that the carer does and, ergo, what their support needs are.

Legislation that has implications for carers is discussed in Chapter 3, however it is worth noting here that in the Care Act (2014) there is recognition that agencies should work closely together to prevent someone having to undergo multiple assessments which may be distressing and confusing (para 6.77). This should prevent the issue of carers having to disclose their details to a stranger on several occasions (once is bad enough). However, having to repeat the same information (which may be distressing information) time and time again is not only frustrating, it takes up valuable time, which comes at a price. There is a lack of respect shown when one is asked again for the details – think about the case study above. What do you think the implications might be if a practitioner carrying out an assessment or a review were to ask both Rob and Sylvia independently: 'So when did you/your husband first start to develop MS?' That information is surely held by the organisation and/or is usually readily available. In order to develop a supportive professional relationship with carers and the person in receipt of care, the above question is unlikely to indicate a good start (Dyke, 2016).

# Carers and identity

So what is the identity of carers? Caring is a weighted concept. If we read online or in a newspaper of a 'grandfather of five' or a 'young mother', immediately pictures form in our minds of who or what that person will be and, based on our own experiences, a pre-judgement is made. That judgement may well be completely removed from reality and is a picture derived from one's own particular background and experiences, which may have no basis in the experiences of others. For example, as a researcher and a carer, I have been privileged to interview many carers over the years. One of the first mistakes I made was to assume I understood their situation and that I would be able to relate to it. While this is, and was certainly true for *some* aspects of the care-giving experience, for others it was so far off the mark as to be naïve. Yes I was, and still am, a carer but I have the benefit of a privileged academic and professional education, with the financial benefits that brings about. I am physically healthy, have a partner, and we own our house in a pleasant area with access to services. I have a steady income, regular holidays and lots of support. The arrogance I displayed when I imagined I would relate to a carer, who I later found out was a single mother with health needs, surviving on benefits in an area of high deprivation, while caring for three people, still shames me. Yes, there were some aspects of our identities that are vaguely similar, but that is as far as it goes. I now know just how unique each carer's situation is, despite outward appearances. Following that early experience, I vowed I would never attempt to claim I understand what 'caring' is. In this book I attempt to highlight aspects that are worthy of further consideration, but I do not have the arrogance to assume I understand the reality for individual carers, and I would urge all those working with carers to be mindful of making similar assumptions. Think of your own situation as a student or an employee and those of others in your cohort or team. There will invariably be differences in age, gender, background, hopes, dreams and aspirations, that make comparisons difficult.

Regardless of my own 'epiphany', however, there is a general societal consensus as to who, or what, constitutes being a 'carer' and indeed many other 'identities'. How do we construct what it is to be a carer?

## Practical **task**

Think about the following words – take them at 'face value' and write down, or draw (be as creative as you like!) what the words mean for you. Don't spend too long thinking about it.

» Mother

» Lawyer

» Teenager

» Airline cabin crew attendant

» Musician

» Scientist

Next, ask a colleague to do the same. Chances are, I imagine, that there will be some similarities – the smartly dressed, well-groomed cabin crew attendant, the wild-haired scientist, for example – but how, and where, do we form these images in our minds, and how closely linked to reality are they? Have you portrayed the people behind the words as either male or female? Black or white? Young or old?

Consider the same newspaper report: if we read of an incident involving a carer aged 35 for example, the word 'carer' in this instance may be taken by many to denote an employment status. Note, I do not use the word 'professional' as despite being a key component in multidisciplinary working, paid carers may not believe that they are seen by others as professionals.

The situation is much the same with family carers. They are a vital part of the team supporting and empowering the cared-for person, and yet in any interprofessional arena or meeting, their views and perspectives are unlikely to be given equal status to others. The issue of identity is further muddled as few carers identify themselves as such. The public perception of carers is generally that of low-paid workers who carry out a range of personal care tasks. Take the case study above for example: Sylvia may not consider herself to be a carer. Sylvia identifies herself as a wife, a mother and a daughter. The imperceptible nature of her caring role, which has increased as Rob's health and well-being have declined and, as her Mother has aged and become more forgetful, has meant that under these circumstances Sylvia is less likely to consider herself as a carer, as opposed to someone whose partner has been suddenly impaired as the result of a road accident, for example.

If being a professional is linked to pay and status then it is worth considering that in order to obtain Carer's Allowance, carers need to be providing care for a minimum of 35 hours a week. This benefit is only payable for one cared-for person. Remember the example above, when I was attempting to compare my situation to a single mother who cared for three people (two of her children had severe learning difficulties, and her mother had dementia). Although Sylvia is providing care for both her husband and her mother, she would only be able to claim for one person. The rate (as at September 2017) is £65.20 per week, that equates to less than £2.00 per hour if 35 hours of care per week is provided. The qualification of only funding care for one person is also a complete anomaly. Who makes such a decision? Presumably, Sylvia's mother is seen to be too old and, in my instance, one child is seen as less worthy than the other and the older adult. The fact that Carer's Allowance is such a low amount, coupled with the fact that it is only payable for one person, may be seen as further evidence of the value the State places on the worth of carers. Carer's Allowance is approximately 25 per cent of the minimum wage, and is the lowest rate for any income replacement benefit (Rummery, 2016). For Sylvia, as with many other carers, there is more than one person with support needs – her husband and her mother. This obviously means more needs to be met, but may also mean that the carer is dealing with more than one support agency and many professionals. On a practical level, consider how that might be managed: most people can relate to taking time off from work waiting at home for a delivery, or a repair to a household appliance, and the frustration felt when that fails to materialise at the set time. Now, imagine if you have that situation, waiting for professionals to arrive to assess or review the needs of an individual. Or if you have to accompany your loved one to an appointment, only to be kept waiting for several hours, then multiply that if you are caring for more than one person. Meetings regarding carers and the person for whom care is received invariably take place during office hours, and professionals are generally unable, in my personal experience, to be able to convene or attend a meeting before 10am or after 4pm. The effect on carers who are trying to balance caring with employment is huge. While going into work late or finishing early may be a possibility, taking an hour (or longer if travelling time is accounted for) away from work at 11am may be less of a possibility.

Caring, however, does have an enormous impact on other aspects of a carer's life. The current political and cultural context in which local authority social services operate within the UK ensures that 'best value' and 'cost effectiveness' are never far from the agenda. Of course, money worries are a major concern for many people, not just carers. However, many carers do have additional demands on their often meagre finances.

We know that carers are less likely to be employed full-time, which has ongoing implications for savings and pension allocation so, for a starting point, their income is likely to be lower than others' in society. This is put against the fact that expenditure is likely to be higher so, to put it crudely, there is less money coming in to the household and more going out.

Using the case study of Sylvia and Rob above, we know that Rob has continence issues. As well as the additional practical time needed to be spent on this, there is also a financial implication as this places extra pressure on the couple's washing machine and tumble dryer, both of which need replacing more frequently than one would normally expect. There is the additional cost of washing powder and conditioner, along with higher electricity bills.

Another fairly basic fact taken from the case study above is that Rob gets through a lot of underwear. He is conscious of the potential for body odour and is keen for Sylvia to purchase body sprays, soaps and aftershave to try and counteract this. Again, this seems trivial, but when money is tight these extra expenses may tip the balance between carers and families coping and struggling financially.

It is not usually the major crises that impact on carers, but rather the smaller day-to-day issues seen by many as insignificant. These build up and have huge potential to have a major impact on carers' physical and emotional health. For some carers money is likely to be less of an issue; for example, if caring is short-term and the person for whom care is being provided has an income or may live 'independently' and perhaps even has a pension or savings in their own right, there may be less of a demand on carers financially – as stated earlier, carers and caring situations are complex and no two are the same. Carers are individuals and their circumstances are unique. Practitioners need to be aware that carers may want to discuss their finances in private. One of my early mistakes as a social worker was to attempt to complete a financial assessment with an older man in receipt of home care services from the local authority while his daughter was present. She extricated herself with a very polite reminder that 'Dad is very private about his income, and I don't think I should be here now' – a salutary reminder about not making assumptions based on one's own experiences of family life, and still a lesson I remember decades later. Carers, like the people in receipt of care, need to be given the option to discuss such matters in private, and as a young eager social worker this was something I failed to remember.

As you may imagine, the details regarding welfare benefits are invariably complex. They depend on income, age and other income and benefits along with, in some cases, interpretation and, in all cases, knowledge of welfare benefits.

For practitioners, as discussed in Chapter 2 it is worth remembering that carers' centres can be useful sources of information and frequently offer benefits advice and guidance. Also, referrals may be made by staff at carers' centres to welfare benefits advisers. A basic inclusion in any practitioner's 'tool kit' is information about services for carers. Again, this sounds quite basic but having such informa-tion to hand – for example, current leaflets that provide information regarding services, and contact details – saves time in the long run, may be helpful and is an indicator that you as a professional have actually thought about the situation before arriving.

Remember that accurate recording and communication are again the key. If every professional involved in a situation gives out the same information, there may be a downside – that is, the carer/person in receipt of care/family may be likely to feel overwhelmed.

This discussion is two-fold when it comes to carers and identity. First, are carers a part of a homogenous social entity to which people feel they belong? Knowles et al (2016) carried out research exploring the needs of carers of people with long-term conditions. They found that carers would frequently draw on comparisons with other carers, particularly those caring for relatives who were more dependent. This was used as a way of explaining their reluctance to define themselves as carers. Additionally, they reported how carers resisted adopting the label 'carer' because of their concerns about the cared-for relative, and how it could make them feel in terms of their own identity. Few carers want to be seen as different, to stand out.

Caring is impacted on in many ways by broader socio-political ideologies that influence the ways in which people and groups are perceived. Broader forces, such as the continuing rise of neoliberal politics and economics and various forms of oppressive behaviour, including xenophobia also fuelled by the emergence of 'populist' movements (Moffitt, 2016), have resulted in unexpected political triumphs and gains (for example, Trump in America and Le Pen in France). In addition, the (almost ubiquitous) Islamophobic rhetoric (Henry, 2018) espoused by many in government, both here and overseas, operate within the broad base of identity politics (Kenny, 2004), and such movements speak to the dangers of 'othering'. To include people solely in broad categories such as 'Muslim' (Tarsin, 2015), 'Chav' (Jones, 2012), 'carer' or 'adult with dementia' is problematic (Bartlett and O'Connor, 2010). How we define people has implications for negating personal identity and focusing solely on one element of people's lives. When such actions take place within a context of austerity, such simplistic representations are more likely to have a disproportionate *negative* impact on the most vulnerable in society, including those giving and receiving care. Carers and those in receipt of care are often seen to occupy a one-dimensional space, possessing a one-dimensional identity, and use resources unfairly. Such attitudes are often based, as we have already seen, on simplistic assertions that equate economic activity with a 'couldn't-care-less' attitude, without due regard for the realities of caring and the ways it limits economic activity for carers and those cared-for.

## Carers' adjustment to their change in identity

The impact of the lived experience of being a carer is enormous and is an ongoing challenge for carers and for those people for whom they care.

Being a carer means, for most people, a change in their roles and in their relationship with the person for whom they are providing care. This may not necessarily mean a negative change. As we observed earlier, for some people their lives were shaped and positively enriched by the opportunities that caring presented. Caring can be rewarding and strengthening, leading to new skill acquisition and a sense of purpose (Brooke, 2016). The discussion in Chapter 2 noted the presence of reciprocal care and discussed the mutually beneficial and supportive relationships that exist between the 'carer' and the 'cared-for'. They are not binary distinct terms.

In terms of carers' identity however, the change in role associated with being a carer may initially be seen as a loss, that notion of one's own taken-for-granted future no longer existing as well as the future of the person in receipt of care. Future plans, hopes and dreams may be denied. The imperceptible nature of such change may be difficult for carers to articulate and could be seen as corrosive, with perhaps the gradual loss of autonomy coupled with an acceptance of the challenges as a status quo.

For practitioners working with families where there is a carer it is important to remember and acknowledge that they are only joining them partway through a journey that started long before the practitioner became involved, and which will more than likely continue long after they have moved on to work with other families. Thus, the major long-term effects of caring are not always noted by the practitioners, who may be expecting carers to articulate this, or even noted by the carers themselves. For some carers their caring journey has been identified as one of 'shame' or 'guilt'. Cherry et al (2017) found this to be particularly the case with carers of people with long-term mental health conditions. Similarly, carers of people with eating disorders experienced shame, guilt and stigma (Treasure and Todd, 2016) and carers who are not able to live close to the person for whom they care also report feelings of guilt (Metzel, 2016). Grief reactions associated with guilt and exhaustion are frequently reported in the literature, particularly when caring for people with dementia. Conflicts about responsibility and decision-making for, and on behalf of, the cared-for person abound. Carers do experience anger, guilt, stigma, stress and feelings of selfishness especially when taking some time for themselves, whether through the use of respite services or short breaks and by understanding this, valuable insights for practitioners to work in an holistic and empathetic way is gained.

Many carers do however recognise the identity of 'carer' and understand and are able to articulate how unsustainable their constant involvement is. They acknowledge they are on the brink of 'burning out' (Ireland, 2016) and may look to practitioners for answers.

## Reflective **task**

Using the information in this chapter and your own personal and professional background, consider the following situations. Who do you think might be 'the carer' and what does the situation tell you about the potential for carers to become overwhelmed and 'burnt out':

» a daughter who cares for her father who has dementia and is known to be verbally abusive;

» a 15-year-old boy who cares for his mother, who is a single parent and has severe anxiety stress and panic attacks;

» an 89-year-old widower, who cares for his 56-year-old son who has Down's syndrome;

» a married couple in their 50s – he has epilepsy, while she has a visual impairment. They provide care for each other.

In the earlier case study, Sylvia states that caring for Rob is her duty, that she promised 'in sickness and in health' and sees this as the promise she made to Rob on their wedding day. Such views and situations aren't uncommon with an ageing population.

Caring is not limited to age, context or location. Having looked at the case study of Sylvia and Rob it is now time to turn attention to a situation involving carers of children and babies.

# Caring for children and babies

In general parents expect to care and provide for their offspring throughout their childhood and beyond, however, with pressures on the health service and the survival beyond infancy of babies and children with very complex medical conditions, we can see that family members are often expected to provide medical and physical care 'above and beyond' what would have been expected 20 years ago.

The unpredictability of survival for many premature infants leads to a situation where parents are just grateful that they have made it and do not question their own emotional and physical abilities to provide care on a huge scale. Serious illnesses and complex health needs are now being met by family members who use medical procedures in their own homes, usually unassisted by 'professionals', to keep their children safe and well. This is a situation that is unlikely to have existed even ten years ago.

Frequently the tasks of caring are commonly assumed to be unskilled (Webb and Tossell, 1999), yet few would dispute that some level of care provision needs a very high level of commitment, skill and awareness.

The campaign 'I'm not a nurse, but ....' (Well Child, 2015) highlights some of the issues parents of children with complex physical needs face on a daily basis. The medical interventions provided by parents include 'peg' feeding, giving intravenous antibiotics, and managing and delivering complex medical procedures for which they have often had limited training, coupled with the associated emotional, physical and financial costs to families by so doing. Care can be intensive and frequent – several times a day and night. Given the complexity of such interventions, the sense of responsibility is enormous. Parents are unlikely to ask for or receive, or even have, available friends or relatives to stand in for a few hours. Remember Sylvia's scenario? Her daughter would come and stay with her husband while she visited her mother. Would she have been so willing to do this if there was a chance of her father choking or having a seizure? Despite this, there are examples in the literature of people with complex health and medical needs, who would once have been hospitalised for a period of time, now being sent home to be cared for by their family (Ward-Griffin and McKeever, 2000).

For carers, symptoms associated with intense or extreme caring include depression, feeling isolated, exhaustion and loneliness (Bevans and Sternberg, 2012). A small amount of stress may be good for us, but the enduring level of the day-to-day 'grind' of such extreme caring may lead to carers being unable to continue, and becoming physically and emotionally unwell themselves. Small problems become insurmountable. The inability to make decisions on very small matters, for example, whether to choose tea or coffee, let alone make important decisions about care-providers becomes impossible. Such intense pressure, coupled with forgetfulness associated with stress and poor sleep, may lead to a situation whereby dangerous practice is occurring. Taking those elements into consideration when carrying out tasks, which in the past would have been the role of trained medical professionals, poses a very worrying situation. We know mistakes are made when medical staff become tired. What about the implications for the care of some very poorly children when parents are expected (and never asked) to deliver 24-hour care?

The negative impact of shift work and long hours (12+) on the medical profession, coupled with issues for patient safety has been well documented in the literature – see, for example, Meghji et al (2015) and Pryce (2016) – and are elsewhere in this text.

The juggling and multitasking that carers are routinely expected to do (and expect to do?) may be phenomenal. If there are other family members that need support and attention (other children, older parents for example) as well as pressures of work, or of just existing, clothes needing to be washed, shopping purchased, meals prepared and bills paid, at the very least, this becomes an Herculanean task. Regarding finances, take for example long-term parent-carers, it is possible to see that they are more likely to be in financial hardship than other 'groups' of carers. Few nurseries and primary schools offer 'wrap round' care that can meet the needs of children with severe learning and/or physical disabilities. The onus is on parents to provide care after school and during school holidays as well as be able to meet and attend appointments relating to their child. This has longer term implications as well: if carers, generally women, have not been part of the labour market for years, there are implications for their own pension and savings.

Asking for help and support may seem, for some, like an admission of guilt and inability to cope. When one's whole identity is consumed by the role of carer it may be difficult for family members to even attempt to raise their heads above the parapet and recognise that other people's lives do not exist along similar trajectories.

Carers may become 'routinised' and begin to normalise their experiences as a way of beginning to make some sense of the path their lives are following. With no other obvious options, or when the alternatives are unclear, requesting assistance may be even more untenable.

# Respite/Short break care

Given the examples discussed above, one suggestion for mitigating some of the difficulties experienced by family carers, particularly with regard to exhaustion and pressure, may be to utilise short breaks or 'respite' services for the person with care and support needs. Such care may be an answer for some people, however, this is not without its own problems. First a suitable location has to be found (with a vacancy available), the cared-for person has to want to (or be persuaded to) go there and then there are the physical practicalities: the transportation of drugs, equipment, clothes and accessories, for what may be only a one-night stay.

The cost of getting there, petrol and time, the enduring worry many carers feel when their loved one is in a short break/respite facility, coupled with the aftermath of dealing with an unsettled relative who may be angry and resentful on return to the family home, all adds to the pressure. Even while their loved one is in respite there may be no 'respite' for the carer. The advances of technology mean that people are contactable 24-hours-a-day 7-days-a-week, and an immediate response is often required. If stories of people using their mobile phones to call home and speak to their parent or carer on an hourly basis when at respite are to be believed, even the most 'gold standard' respite facility may offer little in the way of a break from the caring role.

Then there is the financial cost, together with all associated paperwork: risk assessments also need to be undertaken, papers signed, responsibility allocated, and instructions given. The fact that carers may not be present does not mean they stop 'caring' – far from it. The all-encompassing sense of duty, responsibility, anxiety and worry all combine to make the experience of organising and relying on short break facilities outside of the home a major level of concern that may be difficult for carers to live with.

Practitioners who work with family carers and may advocate for the use of short breaks need to be mindful that they are not seen as a panacea for every situation. For many parent-carers, the opportunity for their child with care and support needs to access a respite facility for one or two nights offers them an opportunity to devote time to siblings. This may be seen as a welcome event and eagerly anticipated, however in reality may develop into a military operation, with the aim to 'have fun at all costs' – the parents themselves may be totally exhausted and would really prefer to lie in a hot bath in a dark room for a couple of hours.

Even with the use of short breaks, opportunities for spontaneity may not exist for carers. Pressures of family life, coupled with housing, financial and employment issues mean that for many carers', relationships become a struggle. Parents of children who have a disability are at greater risk than other parents/carers in terms of the quality of their relationship and are more likely to have higher stress levels (Parkes et al, 2011). Of course there are other ways for both the carer and the cared-for person to obtain a break from the day-to-day routine. As noted in the previous chapter, personalisation and individual budgets offer, in theory, a variety of choice and an individualised approach to needs and these may be utilised in a variety of formats and settings.

What then might practitioners do to support families, carers and the 'whole family' as identified in the Care Act (2014)? First, it is necessary to have an understanding of the fact that carers do not exist in a vacuum – the stigmatising nature of society and the lack of worth generally placed on the lives of people who need support in a variety of ways above the accepted 'norm' (and who is to say what that is at any one time?) impacts on carers. The slow 'drip-drip-drip' of prejudice, discrimination and intolerance intensifies and becomes an almost integral part of people's stories and identities. Relatively simple activities, such as going out for a meal, take on a different hue when the restaurant has to be contacted in advance to see if they are truly accessible. The stress of the unknown, in terms of the person for whom care is given, unpredictability, coupled with the unplanned and unwanted (negative) attention by members of the public, in addition to financial cost and difficulties that may exist in transport to reach the desired location, all weigh heavily on the shoulders of some carers, so much so that it becomes too much to attempt. If Sylvia and Rob, in the case study discussed above, were to use the train they need to make contact in advance to ensure ramps are available. They have to arrive at the station early. When they are on the train, the accessible space for Rob's wheelchair is next to the toilet and Sylvia has to stand. Worlds become smaller and opportunities fewer so that to participate in what the majority of people would not give a second thought to is untenable.

This chapter has focused on a case study to highlight relevant points of interest. Continuing with some of these key issues, including regarding carer identity and the relationship with professionals, the following chapter will explore challenges brought about by caring in a multi-professional arena and debate to what extent carers are truly partners in care.

## Taking it further

1. For more information regarding I'm not a nurse watch www.youtube.com/watch?v=9mNlYDBTP_Y

2. For issues related to multiple sclerosis and care, the following research paper provides an interesting discussion regarding the impact on family members. Bowen, C, MacLehose, A and Beaumont, J G (2011) Advanced multiple sclerosis and the psychosocial impact on families. *Psychology and Health, 26*(1): 113–27.

3. The findings from this paper include issues of self-identity of parent-carers caring for a child with complex health needs. Wang, K W K and Barnard, A (2008) Caregivers' experiences at home with a ventilator-dependent child. *Qualitative Health Research, 18*(4): 501–8.

# References

Bartlett, R and O'Connor, D (2010) *Broadening the Dementia Debate: Towards Social Citizenship.* Bristol: Policy Press.

Bevans, M F and Sternberg, E M (2012) Caregiving burden, stress, and health effects among family caregivers of adult cancer patients. *JAMA, 307*(4): 398–403.

Bowen, C, MacLehose, A and Beaumont, J G (2011) Advanced multiple sclerosis and the psychosocial impact on families. *Psychology and Health,* 26(1): 113–127.

Brooke, J (2016) Caring for patients with dementia. *Nursing in Practice, 89*: 68–71.

Care Alliance Ireland (2016) The Wisdom of Family Carers. *Care Alliance Ireland Discussion Paper Series*.

Cherry, M G, Taylor, P J, Brown, S L, Rigby, J W and Sellwood, W (2017) Guilt, shame and expressed emotion in carers of people with long-term mental health difficulties: a systematic review. *Psychiatry Research, 249*: 139–51.

Dyke, C (2016) *Writing Analytical Assessments in Social Work*. St Albans: Critical Publishing.

Floyd, F J and Gallagher, E M (1997) Parental stress, care demands, and use of support services for school-age children with disabilities and behavior problems. *Family Relations, 46*(4): 359–71.

Hayden, M F and Goldman, J (1996) Families of adults with mental retardation: stress levels and need for services. *Social Work, 41*(6): 657–67.

Henry, D (2018) *Voices of Modern Islam: What it Means to be Muslim Today*. London: Jessica Kingsley Publishers.

Jones, O (2012) *Chavs: The Demonization of the Working Class*. London and New York: Verso Books.

Kenny, M (2004) *The Politics of Identity: Liberal Political Theory and the Dilemmas of Difference*. Cambridge: Polity.

Knowles, S, Combs, R, Kirk, S, Griffiths, M, Patel, N and Sanders, C (2016) Hidden caring, hidden carers? Exploring the experience of carers for people with long-term conditions. *Health & Social Care in the Community*, 24(2): 203–13.

Martin, Y, Gilbert, P, McEwan, K and Irons, C (2006) The relation of entrapment, shame and guilt to depression, in carers of people with dementia. *Aging and Mental Health, 10*(2): 101–6.

Meghji, S, Rajan, N and Philpott, J (2015) What does the junior contract mean for me, my patients and the NHS? *Journal of the Royal Society of Medicine*, 108(12): 470.

Mencap (2006) Breaking point: families still need a break. www.mencap.org.uk/sites/default/files/2016-07/Breaking%20Point%20Families_still_need_a_break%202006.pdf [accessed 1 April 2018].

Metzel, D (2016) 563 miles: a matter of distance in long-distance caring by siblings of siblings with intellectual and developmental disabilities. In *Towards Enabling Geographies: 'Disabled' Bodies and Minds in Society and Space* (p 123). London: Routledge.

Moffitt, B (2016) *The Global Rise of Populism: Performance, Political Style, and Representation*. Palo Alto, CA: Stanford University Press.

Parkes, J, Caravale, B, Marcelli, M, Franco, F and Colver, A (2011) Parenting stress and children with cerebral palsy: a European cross-sectional survey. *Developmental Medicine & Child Neurology*, 53(9): 815–21.

Pearlin, L I, Mullan, J T, Semple, S J and Skaff, M M (1990) Caregiving and the stress process: an overview of concepts and their measures. *The Gerontologist*, 30(5): 583–94.

Pryce, C (2016) Impact of shift work on critical care nurses. *Canadian Journal of Critical Care Nursing, 27*(4): 17–21.

Roper, S O, Allred, D W, Mandleco, B, Freeborn, D and Dyches, T (2014) Caregiver burden and sibling relationships in families raising children with disabilities and typically developing children. *Families, Systems, & Health*, 32(2): 241–6.

Rummery, K (ch 14) in Bochel, H and Powell, M (eds) (2016) *The coalition government and social policy: Restructuring the welfare state*. Bristol: Policy Press.

Shah, A J, Wadoo, O and Latoo, J (2010) Psychological distress in carers of people with mental disorders. *British Journal of Medical Practitioners*, 3(3): a327.

Tarsin, A (2015) *Being Muslim: A Practical Guide*. Davie, FL: Sandala Incorporated.

Todd, S and Jones, S (2003) 'Mum's the word!': maternal accounts of dealings with the professional world. *Journal of Applied Research in Intellectual Disabilities*, 16(3): 229–44.

Treasure, J and Todd, G (2016) Interpersonal maintaining factors in eating disorder: skill sharing interventions for carers. In *Bio-Psycho-Social Contributions to Understanding Eating Disorders* (pp 125–37). New York: Springer.

Wang, K W K and Barnard, A (2008) Caregivers' experiences at home with a ventilator-dependent child. *Qualitative Health Research*, 18(4): 501–8.

Ward-Griffin, C and McKeever, P (2000) Relationships between nurses and family caregivers: partners in care? *Advances in Nursing Science*, *22*(3): 89–103.

Webb, R and Tossell, D (1999) *Social Issues for Carers: Towards Positive Practice*. London: Arnold.

Well Child (2015) #notanurse_but. www.wellchild.org.uk/supporting-you/notanurse_but/ [accessed 1 April 2018].

Williams, V and Robinson, C (2000) *In Their Own Right: The Carers Act and Carers of People with Learning Disabilities*. Bristol: Policy Press.

Williams, V and Robinson, C (2001) 'He will finish up caring for me': people with learning disabilities and mutual care. *British Journal of Learning Disabilities*, *29*(2): 56–62.

# Chapter 5 | Professionals and caring

*At last, carers will be given the same recognition, respect and parity of esteem with those they support. Historically, many carers have felt that their roles and their own well-being have been undervalued and under-supported. Now we have a once in a lifetime opportunity to be truly acknowledged and valued as expert partners in care.*

(Dame Philippa Russell, Chair, Standing Commission on Carers,
Department of Health, 2014)

To what extent are carers actually valued as 'expert partners in care' as Dame Russell suggested the Care Bill, now the Care Act (UK Government, 2014), intended? This chapter looks at the idea of partnership, and how carers are viewed in a multi-professional arena by (other) professionals, by the person for whom care is provided, and how they view themselves. Examining what is meant by being 'a professional', and being 'professional', this chapter will examine some of the common myths and perceptions associated with care provision, and highlight some of the advantages and disadvantages associated with such. Using the four models or 'ideal types of the response of service agencies to carers' proposed by Twigg and Atkin (1994, p 11) this chapter will consider the ways that carers are viewed by professionals in the UK in the twenty-first century.

Implicit within the Care Act (UK Government, 2014a) is the importance of partnership, and the idea of being an expert, let alone an expert partner, may be seen by some as being an attractive one. It can be flattering to be asked for advice and guidance by those less experienced than oneself. Taking 'expert' as meaning a person who is very knowledgeable about, or skillful in a particular area, one can see that this would apply to many carers. Carers often have unique knowledge of a particular situation, and know how, and when, to intervene or to offer appropriate and timely support. The skills needed to apply this particular knowledge may also be unique to that individual, and are in many cases skills that have been acquired through many years of hands-on experience.

## Partners in care

Some organisations and hospital trusts explicitly have 'partners in care schemes' where 'expert' carers work closely to advise such organisations about best practice in working with carers. Seen in some mental health services and linked to carers organisations, the partnerships are a valuable way of multi-professional working and offering advice and feedback to support the work that is carried out. Carers who are expert partners often find their role is to act as a 'critical friend' and offer advice and support as well as monitoring progress, through their accumulated expertise. Such arrangements strengthen partnerships and help to develop networks between the carers organisation and the hospital trust (for more information see the Carers Trust Triangle of Care https://professionals.carers.org/triangle-care-toolkit/carer-service-user-partners).

Partnership working involving carers is not without its challenges. It may take a strong practical, moral and financial commitment from a variety of different and often powerful individuals and groups, including chief executives, directors and senior managers from health and social care settings, to establish this, and it takes even more commitment to maintain long-term involvement that is not just tokenistic. The support of advocacy groups and carers organisations is vital in developing and maintaining such a partnership. Finding a range of carers representatives of the area in question, who have time and interest, is not an easy option. Partnership with carers should include full involvement in all aspects of the topic under discussion. This may mean designing, exploring and reviewing specific services. It should not be tokenistic: carers should be active in their involvement if partnership is to be attempted and, indeed, if it is deemed to be successful. Having one 'token' carer on a board or merely relying on a brief consultation is not enough. In an expert partnership, carers need to be in an active role and their involvement should be based on a sharing of power. Appropriate financial recompense also needs to be made.

## Reflective **task**

When thinking about how to involve carers in meetings or projects, try to think 'outside the box'.

Different times and different locations are more conducive to some carers for their involvement than others. Some carers may be able to attend a meeting at 9am: however realistically for many it might be better placed late morning when the person for whom they care has gone out, or has had their immediate practical needs met. Likewise, for some carers, evening meetings may be preferable, although again this might need negotiation.

Carers' time is precious; no lunch breaks, bank holidays or paid annual leave, so it is important that, if they are to attend a meeting, it begins promptly and finishes at a pre-arranged time. Practicalities such as making the meeting space accessible and providing affordable parking, with speedy financial recompense for carers' involvement is also needed. Likewise, if comment or opinion is needed on a particular project, it is important that carers have ample time to read, process, and prepare to feed back their thoughts and opinions on the document. Again, none of this is rocket science: good planning, preparation and being clear about what is expected, is, as with most things, key to a successful partnership.

## Practical **task**

Who are 'The Professionals'?

Taking, as an example, a meeting for a young person (age 17) with severe learning difficulties. In this instance the meeting is a transitions (from child to adult services) meeting to discuss future plans and options for that young person.

Those persons listed below are in attendance:

» Head of School Year

» Speech and Language Therapist

» Social Worker (Local Authority Child in Need Team)

» Social Work Student

» Social Worker (Local Authority Vulnerable Adults Team)

» Transitions Adviser

» Residential Care Worker

» Parent

» Classroom Assistant

» Community Learning Disability Nurse

» Psychiatrist

» Young person's advocate

How many of the above do you consider to belong to a profession?

What do you see as defining the role of a profession?

Make a note of this and then ask a colleague to do the same.

Be prepared to share your answers.

When you have answered the above, I imagine the chances are you would have found some attendees at the meeting easier to identify as professionals than others. For example, a psychiatrist will have undertaken several years of education to achieve that status, similarly, speech and language therapy is a degree level entry occupation, as are social work and teaching. The situation becomes more complicated when considering a classroom assistant and a transitions adviser, while not necessarily degree level occupations, those workers may have decades of experience over a newly qualified social worker completing the assessed and supported year of employment (ASYE). This begs the question: are qualifications valued over and above experience when deciding who is to be considered as a professional? If experience and knowledge of the individual's situation are considered to be key, then surely the parent of the young person will come out top in experience stakes?

As a counter balance to this discussion, the opposite of 'professional' is the word 'amateur', seen perhaps as a less attractive option. The notion of 'amateur' implies someone who is not committed and does not 'give their all'. In order to obtain 'professionalism', as many practitioners have found, it may be a case of 'act as if' or 'fake it 'til you make it!'

## Case study example

Charlotte is 21 and a newly qualified social worker, currently undergoing her assessed and supported year of practice (ASYE). Charlotte is, on the whole, enjoying her job but feels that, on occasions, some people she works with make it clear that they would rather have a more experienced colleague. Following discussions in supervision, and reflecting on what may be the reasons for this, Charlotte decides to emulate her mentor's techniques and approach to working with people and hopes to build her own professional style from that. She notices that Katy, her mentor, is polite and friendly, but keeps 'chat' to a minimum and focuses on the job to be done. Katy is very organised and communicates clearly while avoiding jargon, something Charlotte feels she would love to be able to do.

When reflecting on Katy's style of working, Charlotte recalls a long visit she made to meet with a man who had recently been in receipt of care services. When the man asked how she was, Charlotte remembered how she had then proceeded to tell him – in detail – excitedly chatting about her plans for her birthday next week, and the forthcoming trip to London her boyfriend is taking her on. Charlotte initially thought the meeting must have gone well as, Callum, the person for whom care was being provided, told her all about his last trip to London and about the time he went to the Imperial War Museum. Before Charlotte realised it, the meeting had lasted for 90 minutes and she still had not got the basic information she had set out to obtain.

Charlotte realised that she needed to 'perform' more as a professional and less of 'Charlotte the newly qualified, eager to please, social worker'. By doing this, she hoped she would eventually develop the confidence to develop these skills naturally, committed as she was to acting on the imposed self-belief. Charlotte realised that when she had graduated from university part of her thought, that was it – she was a ready-made professional. By seeing her career as more of a marathon than a sprint and being committed to working towards her goals, Charlotte now feels that she is on the path towards achieving this.

# Are carers professionals?

Collaborative working involves different professionals, agencies, the people who use services as well as carers, working, as it says, in a collaborative way. Multi-professional working, interprofessional working and collaborative working are all terms used interchangeably. For many carers, multi-professional working can seem to take place without their involvement, or at the expense of their time with the given professionals (SCIE, 2009). The views and wishes of carers should feed into policy, learning and practice and add to the body of knowledge about the individual in receipt of care. This needs not to be tokenistic. Collaboration has many benefits – for example, it is seen as a way of reducing costs and streamlining efficiency. Evidence suggests that working inter-professionally improves outcomes for both carers and the person in receipt of care (see, for example, Hammick et al, 2007).

Working in partnership with carers to ensure that their voice (as well as the voice of the person in receipt of care) is heard, may be complex, however, it is key to successful collaboration. Those people who are the ones performing a role on a regular basis are usually the best placed to understand it. Talking to carers can often produce information about the services being provided, or received, that you may not get in any other way. Responsibility for supporting the needs of carers does not just come from one profession, or from one sector within that profession. Rather, a multi-agency approach involving health, education (particularly relevant when looking at the experiences of young carers – see Chapter 7), local authorities, and other agencies, as appropriate, is called for.

Pay and status are two of the most recognisable characteristics of what makes someone a professional. However, carers are unpaid (with the exception of Carer's Allowance) and the role is not generally seen as a high status one. The recent debate regarding recompense for those paid carers, when working in residential settings overnight on a sleep-in shift, have brought this debate into focus. Companies and charities that provide care have traditionally provided a flat rate for a sleep-in shift, generally in the region of £30. For some time now it appears that there has been a realisation that the national minimum wage (£7.50 for over-25-year-olds in England, December 2017) needs to be paid for these hours. This has huge implications for these organisations. Critics are suggesting that it is the failure of the government to adequately fund social care that now risks devastating the care sector and not workers requesting a legal wage. The debate regarding back-pay to those employees who have provided sleep-in shifts in the past continues, with the government now announcing that employers will be able to opt into a new social-care compliance scheme. This will give them a year to determine what they owe to workers who have previously carried out sleep-ins and will be backed by advice from Her Majesty's Revenue and Customs (HMRC).

Consider the same scenario applied to family carers: if, as estimated by a recent report (Yeandle and Buckner, 2007), carers save the government £132 billion per year, this figure would rise dramatically once the basic minimum wage is included for weekly 'pay' let alone if sleep-in pay was included. Carer's Allowance is £62.70 per week (2017/ 2018). In order to claim this allowance one has to be providing care for at least 35 hours per week. On a purely practical basis this equates to £1.92 per hour. Additionally, there are certain conditions applied to this, if the basic minimum wage was paid for 35 hours per week then a payment of £262 would be required to be made. Imagine the financial implications of this and also if family carers were paid by the State for overnight care.

For many, the experience of providing care to a friend or relative becomes more than simply a job. As the years go by and the caring experience becomes extended, a 'career' develops (albeit one in which there is little pay, no career enhancement, no holidays, and a career in which the terms and conditions would be seen by most other employees as unfavourable). Reading this, one may wonder why people continue to provide daily care for their friends and relatives that may be both physically and emotionally exhausting. Reasons why people do care are discussed in Chapter 3. However, in summary here, I believe that the very act of caring helps to define humanity at its most giving, supportive, empathetic and nurturing. It is important to note that not all caring is one way; caring needs to be seen as relational while taking into account the visceral nature of our human bodies. While recognising it as a universal activity which can be incredibly rewarding it is still, in many circumstances, a way of life that many struggle with as it may develop gradually and continue for decades.

Parent-carers of children and adults with impairments tend to provide care for the longest period of time. Other caring scenarios tend to be more short-term: people move in and out of caring scenarios during their lives.

No one agency or body of professionals should have the monopoly of providing for, or understanding, the needs of family carers. Likewise, agencies need to work closely together (including input from carers and those they care for) to ensure an holistic approach to the issues that are faced.

# Imposter syndrome

In discussing the question, are carers professionals?, it is useful to consider for a moment 'imposter syndrome'. Imposter syndrome is, in essence, when an individual suffers foundationless thoughts of incompetence or inadequacy when considering their own abilities. Feelings of fraudulence and a lack of confidence in one's ability (Chapman, 2015), can often abound with carers. Often linked to low self-esteem and feelings of being inadequate, individuals doubt their own skills and fear the judgement of their peers. Many carers may hold stereotypical views of who, or what, a carer is and then believe they fall short of that. Peer support and a sense of connection to people and services is crucial to help manage the feelings of imposter syndrome (Chapman, 2015; Ramsey and Brown, 2017) and yet, for many carers, the isolation they experience as part of their caring role precludes them from that option. Practitioners have an important role to play as they may be best placed to support carers to re-navigate their self-image (Ramsey and Brown, 2017) and by so doing may include a sense of their role and their ability to provide high level successful care.

Of course it is not just carers who may feel they are imposters in their role. Practitioners may attribute their successes to luck, or being in the right place at the right time, as opposed to directly being linked to their own actions. Again, peer support from colleagues and regular supervision may be key to developing higher self-esteem and self-belief.

## Personal **reflection**

I can still remember the nagging doubts I had when I approached my daughter's school for the first Christmas assembly and the feeling that I shouldn't be there – they (other parents) appeared on the surface more competent, and in control of their situation (and emotions) than I could ever imagine I would be. They seemed to know each other and had an easy relationship with the teaching staff, whereas I felt awkward, out of place and tearful, and that (exhausting) feeling of acting or pretending to be a 'grown up' in that situation has never really left me.

# Twigg and Atkin's model of caring

When exploring the role of carers in society it is interesting to explore a 'seminal' work regarding typologies. The role of carers, and the response of agencies, was portrayed in 1994 by Julia Twigg and Karl Atkin as being one that occurred in one of four distinct models. These models exemplify an 'ideal' type of response by agencies, and while it is important to recognise that they are not mutually exclusive, it is useful to have an understanding of some of the ways that professionals may 'typically' respond to, and work with, the involvement of carers. There is much to be learned from the ways organisations interact with carers and the person in receipt of care. The 'client group' is also instrumental in considering the way carers were seen by, and worked with, professionals. This was, therefore, influential in determining the professional response to carers. The four types are described as being:

> » carers as resources;
>
> » carers as co-workers;
>
> » carers as co-clients;
>
> » carers superseded.

Viewing carers as a resource in essence refers to the overriding idea of social care where the majority of support to meet an individual's needs comes from the 'informal sector' (Twigg and Atkin, 1994, p 12). Such informal care is accepted and unquestioned by professionals and, as a consequence of this, carers are viewed as a (generally) free resource to be drawn upon as, and when, needed.

The internalised notion of 'family' and the taken for granted assumptions that arise from these notions support the idea that care is a given in any relationship where one person has needs that they may have difficulty in meeting without some sort of support or involvement from others. Carers within this model are seen more broadly, and the focus may be on more than one individual – they are in many instances seen as a taken for granted 'free' service. The assumption is that they will provide care and support. Within this model, centre stage is always taken by the person in receipt of care. The (often) unspoken assumption is that formal ie paid care services, only become involved when an 'informal' family carer does not exist.

Twigg and Atkin's typology of carers as co-workers, the second in the four models of care, is seen as an indication of the ways agencies work alongside carers, with support threaded through, and help and support drawn from other family members and friends. While similar to the 'carer as resource' model noted above, the 'carer as co-worker' model assumes centre stage for the person with care needs, but this model also highlights the well-being of the carer. This may be seen in purely instrumental terms: if a carer's well-being, or morale, dips then they may be less able to deliver high quality care and may even be unable to continue with their caring role. This, the second part of Twigg and Atkin's framework, maintains a focus on the person whose needs are being met. (Twigg and Atkin refer to this person as the disabled person. I would suggest widening this to include all those in receipt of care services – for example, people who misuse substances and therefore may have care needs.) The 'carer as co-worker' model recognises the importance of the carer in the life of the person in receipt of care, particularly in relation to morale building. This model focuses on the instrumental value of the carer, recognising it as a means to an end. The assumption is that carers choose to provide care, and by supporting them to do this, high quality care is provided for the person in receipt of care. It is suggested that this definition of carers is wider than the 'carers as a resource' model. The typology of carers as resources and co-workers was noted by Manthorpe et al in 2003 as models that best matched professionals' understanding of the role of the needs of carers. While Twigg and Atkin's framework was constructed over two decades ago, the categorisation still has much to offer when considering the ways that carers are viewed by professionals in the twenty-first century.

With the advent of the Care Act 2014 the third model of care considered seems to be particularly relevant today. Remember the possibility of combined assessments under the Care Act (2014a)? This epitomises the notion of carers as co-clients, of reciprocity and of mutual support and mutual or combined 'needs'. The idea of carers as co-clients, people who both deliver support and need services to support themselves, is particularly aimed at those carers who provide a lot of 'heavy end' caring. The potential for disagreements and conflict between the person in receipt of care and the carer in the traditional sense is recognised in this model. In order for a combined needs assessment to take place both parties must agree to that happening. Both parties need to be provided with an opportunity to speak in private to the assessor. Practitioners may need to set clear parameters when looking at combined assessments of needs – while drawing on the strength of the relationship, it is still important to note they are working with two individuals.

With regard to the carers as co-clients model, carers are seen as being people in need themselves. This model could most usefully be seen as current, given recent legislative changes brought about by the Care Act (2014) where carers are seen as being on an equal basis with those in receipt of care. For Twigg and Atkin this may even be exceeded so the needs of a carer trump the needs of the person for whom they care, with services being provided on the basis of supporting the carer over that of the cared-for person. Use of respite service is a case in point; there is seen to be potential for a conflict of interest between the carer and the person for whom care is provided. Is respite, or a short break in an out of home location, designed to benefit the person in receipt of care, the carer, or both? The key appears to be in who is the recipient of such care; although replacement care, such as a respite break may give the carer a break, it is the adult with care needs who is the recipient of such, and most likely will be recorded in their care and support plan, and budget. The emphasis of the model of carers as co-client highlights these complexities.

Finally, for Twigg and Atkin the model of carers, as superseded, refers to their not being needed due to the notion of the developing and increasing independence of the person in receipt of care. Therefore, the carer gives up caring or is no longer needed to provide care. There are two paths to this final stage in that of superseded carers.

One path leads to the intervention that occurs on behalf of the person in receipt of care. The idea behind this is in terms of maximising the person in receipt of care's independent living skills, and recognising the restrictions placed on people's lives by those family members and friends who are their carers. This model also recognises the imbalance of power between the carer and the cared-for person.

The second path is regarding concern for the carer and their sustainability in their role. With this we might consider an example of care provided by a spouse, perhaps an older couple, where one partner has dementia and is becoming increasingly violent. Taking the morale of the carer seriously within this model, according to Twigg and Atkin, the superseded carer may not at this stage be described as a carer, rather they are seen as 'relatives' or 'friends' without the label of carer.

The majority of help and support that is provided by people in receipt of care comes from family carers. If we see, as some professionals may, that carers are in the category of being 'used' as a resource, does this then perhaps reflect an overwhelming notion society in general has of the 'purpose' of carers?

Obviously these categories are not silos in which to place carers or the response of professionals to working with them. Likewise, they are not fixed and the response of the agency or individual practitioner varies depending on a number of factors, including their role in the hierarchy of that organisation, and the specific needs and diagnosis of the person in receipt of care. For example, Twigg and Atkin's (1994) typology sees front line practitioners as tending to view carers as co-workers, whereas staff on a managerial level view carers through the 'carers as resource' lens, thus seeing them as the most practical and economic way of supporting people with care needs. It would be interesting to explore whether the impact of the financial crisis and the follow-on period of austerity has altered these perspectives in any significant way. Recognising that this model was produced over 20 years ago does not dampen its impact today. It is viewed by many commentators on care, and caring, as seminal in its field. What it does is to provide us with a useful starting point when exploring the relationship between carers and health and social care agencies and professionals.

In order to expand this debate it is important to consider what we mean by 'professionals'. Here the debate goes back even further, making Twigg and Atkin's 1994 framework seem recent!

# Who, or what, is a professional?

Flexner, in a seminal speech in 1915 (2001), debated the issue of what is a professional. Taking social work as an example (still viewed by many as a quasi-profession), Flexner begins by comparing the word 'profession' with its opposite – 'amateur'. He suggests that occupations or roles that were once non-professional have developed into ones that hold professional status. Flexner recognised over 100 years ago that these changes will continue.

If, therefore, we take the raw definitions of a professional as being that of:

» Professional: Engaged in a profession, especially one requiring advanced knowledge or training.

» Professionalism: The body of qualities or features, as competence, skill, etc., characteristic of a profession or professional (Oxford English Dictionary, 2015).

Flexner (1915/2001) can be 'credited' with damaging social work's reputation as a profession because it did not/could not evidence a clear and credible knowledge base, citing medicine as the 'standard bearer' for credibility. That carers tend to be socialised into their role, which many then internalise, appears to be – on the surface – 'good enough' to allow them to be considered as professional. Increasingly associated with professionalism is the idea of financial autonomy, of budget holding and financial or economic prudence. As we have seen in Chapter 3, with the advent of personalisation there comes a relatively new era of budget holding and management by carers – further strengthening their right to professional status perhaps?

## Reflective **task**

Do you think care-giving has a 'clear and credible knowledge base'?

If so, what have you based this on?

If not, why do you think this is?

It may be helpful to debate this with a colleague, each take an opposing view (even if it is not one you hold) and try to debate the merits of your (perhaps imposed) standpoint.

If we take these thoughts and apply them to caring, it may be possible to see that:

» Caring, in many instances, requires advanced knowledge or training (note 'requires' – not always the same as receives).

» Caring within the activities of such, contains a body of qualities and features, combined with evidence of competence and skill.

» Carers have access (albeit often unwillingly) to budgets and have some degree of autonomy in time management – particularly when compared to an office culture.

Just as the ideas around what is a professional are fraught with disagreement and debate, so too is the notion of 'professional values'. Within any exploration on the professionalism of (unpaid) family carers comes the debate around values.

## Practical **task**

Do you think values drawn from one's life differ from those held professionally?

What do you define as your own core values?

Take a moment to write a list of at least five things that you relate to as being your core values.

Now think about your professional role, or your role as a student. Write another list.

Do these lists differ?

Core values are the fundamental beliefs a person has, they guide and shape behaviour, both personal and professional. When I worked through this exercise, I came up with the following list:

My personal core values are (in no particular order): Autonomy, freedom, tolerance, belief in others, and calmness, whereas in a professional sense I would say that, commitment, account-ability, integrity, competence and achievement are values I aspire to.

Categorisation of carers also takes place, notably in the research literature according to two major divisions:

» the needs or diagnosis of the person for whom care is provided;

» the relationship between the carer and person in receipt of care.

Within both these divisions are elements of professionalism and of values.

When considering the first point, we see carers as being defined as being inextricably linked to the experience of being carers for a person with dementia, or carers for a person with multiple sclerosis, or carers for a person with mental health issues for example (Brodaty and Donkin, 2009; Rollero, 2016; Yesufu-Udechuku et al, 2015).

Within the second definition, the emphasis is on the relationship between the two, for example, spousal carers, parent-carers, young carers. In both examples, carers are piv-otal to ensure an appropriate, timely and effective 'service' is provided to the person for whom they care.

Regardless of the definition of and identity given to carers by the typology of care and, as stated in Chapter 2, the lack of homogeneity between carers, descriptions of role and tasks become difficult to identify. Carers generally come to the attention of practitioners due to their relationship with the person in receipt of care and are seen as an adjunct to their role.

The subtle, complex and often specific 'insider' knowledge held by a carer, combined with a wealth and depth of 'practice wisdom', makes it difficult to articulate the extent to which caring is seen as a professional activity. Working with family carers provides practitioners with some insight into understanding in part the role held by them.

# Assessments

What is the role for practitioners when assessing carers in order to establish their needs? Legislation relating to assessments tends to be aspirational – and we might ask what, or where, is the infrastructure needed to support these worthy aspirations?

Given the political and economic climate in twenty-first century Britain the infrastructure needed to support these is unlikely, therefore the aspirations disclosed by carers and noted (and supported?) by practitioners, tend to be rhetorical. Those with statutory responsibility need to satisfy themselves that carers are able and willing to continue to care and are not just paying lip service to it. An overwhelming sense of responsibility is difficult to articulate from a carer's point of view. However, skilled professionals should be able to determine what care is wanted, and needed, as well as their willingness and ability to provide the level of care required. Assessments need to be done properly, and this takes time. While organisational pressures and issues relating to a lack of resources are recognised, it is important that these are not seen as excuses and a rationale for overlooking this fact. This is important and has potential to make a difference to people's lives.

There is recognition for carers within the eligibility outcomes of the Care Act (2014) regarding the impact their caring role has upon their responsibilities to care for children and maintain family and other personal relationships. This may well provide new opportunities for practitioners to be able to intervene positively and gather and provide evidence needed for the provision of services.

Evidence of eligibility for support services from the local authority is required, and carers are entitled to support if they are assessed as having needs that meet the eligibility criteria:

» care for a person who resides in the local authority area;

» accept the charge for services (if there is to be one).

## Case study

Mr Davis (89), a widower, lives alone in a small village in a rural area. He has one daughter, Pauline, a full-time administrator, who lives 15 miles away and who offers him regular support mainly to do with shopping, laundry, meal preparation and some personal care. Mr Davis is becoming increasingly frail and is unsteady on his feet due to his worsening arthritis and deteriorating eyesight.

Under the Care Act 2014, if Pauline and Mr Davis both agree, a combined assessment of their needs could be carried out. Alternatively, for Pauline, a separate carer's assessment would be offered. This would establish how willing and able she is to provide, and continue to provide care to her father.

A carer's assessment would also look at how best to promote Pauline's well-being, and would explore any outcomes she would want to achieve.

**Questions:**

» How would you, as a practitioner, attempt to establish if a combined or separate assessment would be the most appropriate?

» What questions would you ask to satisfy yourself that Pauline was, or was not, willing and able to continue to provide support for her father on a regular basis?

» How would you ensure that there was an opportunity for a private conversation with Mr Davis and Pauline if a combined assessment was agreed?

# Carer's assessment

The Care Act (2014a) brought about a fundamental shift in the way that assessing the needs of carers takes place. Carers are now entitled to an assessment of their needs in their own right. They no longer have to specifically request an assessment. When carrying out an assessment under the Care Act (2014) a key element is exploring 'needs' – that is, those needs of carers and of the people who are in receipt of care and who use services.

Assessment is divided into three stages, namely:

identifying needs;

assessing eligibility;

care planning (Schwehr, 2014).

So, what happens? Obviously not all carers are assessed – not all want to be – and a carer may choose to refuse to have an assessment. This could be down to a myriad of reasons: perhaps because they do not feel that they provide care, they do not want formal acknowledgement of their role as a carer, or they may not want local authority support. In such circumstances local authorities are not required to carry out an assessment.

However, there are many different 'journeys' through the care and assessment process if a carer does want an assessment. Local authorities are organisations that are responsible for public services in a given area. They are public bodies and spend public money. The money local authorities spend comes from a combination of national and local taxes as well as charges to service users. Local authorities have a pivotal role in assessments of carers' needs.

## Beginning an assessment

The following example has been adapted from Feldon (2017) taking account of the case study of Rob and Sylvia in Chapter 4. Remember that Sylvia Twigger is a 58-year-old female who resigned from her full-time job as a retail manager to care for her husband, Rob, who is aged 60 and has multiple sclerosis. It is important to remember that different local authorities have a variety of preferred methods for people to get in touch with them. Some are through telephone calls to a specialised team, known as 'gateways' or 'customer hubs' or 'customer access' teams. These are designed to free up front line staff etc.

In the case of Sylvia and Rob, Sylvia telephoned her local authority two years ago, on the advice of her neighbour. Rob was in agreement with this, as they both recognised that additional help would be necessary.

Sylvia used a telephone number she saw in the library for a 'Customer Access Team' and asked for someone to come and see her and Rob. She briefly explained the circumstances.

After a short discussion, the customer access team adviser concluded that Rob appeared to have needs for care and support and that Sylvia appeared to have needs for support (note the difference) which is, in Care Act terminology, known as an initial assessment at first contact ie the first stage of an assessment. The adviser explained what would happen next, namely that a social worker would be in touch and gave some examples of the types of questions they would be asking. The adviser also said that she would send some information in the post for Rob and Sylvia to read, which would explain what they might expect in terms of timescales, how they might make a complaint if needed, as well as some general information about access to advocacy services.

Two weeks later, Sylvia was contacted by a social worker who arranged an appointment to meet the couple and to carry out an initial assessment. Assessment under the Care Act (2014) should be both an appropriate, and proportionate, assessment which identifies their level of needs. Where appropriate, an assessment may be carried out over the phone or online. However, in this example, a face-to-face visit was arranged following a telephone call to arrange this. Regardless of the format of the assessment, local authorities must ensure that assessors have the skills, knowledge and competence to carry out such an assessment, and Sylvia is relieved to know that a qualified social worker will be visiting them.

# Combined assessments

Rob and Sylvia have decided that they would like to have a combined assessment. Local authorities may combine an assessment of an adult needing care and support, or of a carer, with any other assessment it is carrying out either of that person or another where both the individual and carer agree. One of the main benefits of this is that it will eliminate the authority carrying out two separate assessments when the two assessments are intrinsically linked. Before the visit, the social worker has forwarded a list of areas she will be covering during the assessment. Rob and Sylvia find these really helpful, and begin to think about their responses as well as discussing between themselves their hopes and fears for the future. Paragraph 6.19 of The Care and Support Statutory Guidance (revised 2017) indicates that the carer's assessment must also consider the outcomes that the carer wants to achieve in their daily life, their activities beyond their caring responsibilities, and the impact of caring upon those activities. Rob and Sylvia's discussion leads to them both concluding that Sylvia needs to get out of the house more and follow her own interests. For Sylvia, this discussion and having sight of the proposed questions leads her to think in greater depth about her caring role and responsibilities. For her, ideal outcomes include a wish to join a cake decorating class and to be able to visit the hairdressers once a week.

When carrying out an assessment, practitioners need to be conversational without being overly chatty – a key skill! An assessment needs to be an intervention in itself, so that an individual will benefit from the process itself, no matter what the outcome is.

Assessment is both about needs (in this instance, both Rob's and Sylvia's) and about outcomes. By outcomes, is meant what is needed to maintain or improve the situation. During an assessment, people are encouraged to think about what their needs are, and what outcomes would be needed to improve or maintain the status quo, as well as ways in which these outcomes may be achieved. The assessment showed that Rob's needs came about as a result of his illness, and he is unable to achieve two or more of the outcomes specified in Section 2 (2) of the Care and Support (Eligibility Criteria) Regulations 2014a Act. Consequently, there will be a significant impact on his well-being. Well-being is defined in Section 1 (2) of the Care Act:

(2) 'Well-being', in relation to an individual, means that individual's well-being so far as relating to any of the following:

    (a)    personal dignity (including treatment of the individual with respect);

    (b)    physical and mental health and emotional well-being;

    (c)    protection from abuse and neglect;

    (d)    control by the individual over day-to-day life (including over care and support, or support provided to the individual and the way in which it is provided);

(e)  participation in work, education, training or recreation;

(f)  social and economic well-being;

(g)  domestic, family and personal relationships;

(h)  suitability of living accommodation;

(i)  the individual's contribution to society.

Sylvia's needs came about as a consequence of providing care to Rob. She is unable to achieve two or more of the specified outcomes, therefore there is a significant impact on her well-being.

It is important to note that under the Care Act, an individual's needs must be assessed before eligibility can be determined. When determining whether an adult meets the eligibility criteria, it is important for practitioners to note that any activities under-taken by a carer to meet care and support needs must not be taken into account. Statutory guidance is clear about this: information on the care being provided by a carer can be captured during an assessment, but the eligibility determination must be based solely on the adult's needs, regardless of whether they are met by the carer (SCIE, 2014: www.scie.org.uk/care-act-2014/assessment-and-eligibility/eligibility/files/eligibility.pdf).

Once eligibility was established in the case of Rob and Sylvia, the assessor arranged for a financial assessment to take place. Rob has little in the way of savings and income and his financial resources were deemed to be below the financial limit. A care and support plan was then developed in conjunction with Rob and Sylvia to establish the best way to meet Rob's and Sylvia's needs.

For a more detailed discussion of the components of a needs assessment, please see Feldon (2017). However, for the purposes of providing an understanding of the process or journey that a carer undertakes for an assessment of need, the above example may be useful.

In the example above, a combined assessment was completed. Whether this is a single or a combined assessment, where someone provides, or intends to provide, care for another adult and it appears that the carer may have any level of need for support, local authorities must carry out a carer's assessment.

When assessing, it is important for the assessor to ensure that the feasibility or sustainability of any caring role is a key factor.

Paragraph 6.18 of the UK Government Care and Support Statutory Guidance (revised 2017) states that carers' needs assessments must seek to establish not only the carer's needs for support, but also the *sustainability* of the caring role. Paragraph 6.18 also describes sustainability as including;

» both practical and emotional support which the carer provides to the adult;

» the carer's potential needs for support in the future;

» the ability and the willingness of the carer to continue in that role.

Carers themselves may need support in recognising issues around sustainability, and in knowing and articulating their own needs. Support given to this will be able to assist the assessor to produce a clear rationale for the carer's present and future needs for support and whether the caring relationship appears to be feasible, and one which looks as though it is potentially likely to continue. Empathic and experienced practitioners will be able to draw out nuances and subtleties in their discussions with carers that will help to both understand and facilitate ways of exploring the impact of the caring role on day-to-day life.

As with all good quality assessments the key is in preparation. Research from the Social Care Institute for Excellence (www.scie.org.uk/care-act-2014/assessment-and-eligibility/strengths-based-approach/what-makes-a-good-assessment.asp) has indicated that what people want from an assessment includes the following:

» Flexibility and perceptiveness of any given situation.

» Giving people time to process the information/questions that one may be posing. (This may involve taking extra time, or offering a break if needed to avoid an individual becoming overwhelmed. However, one longer visit in which high quality and useful information is obtained is worth it as opposed to having to follow up because you hadn't obtained sufficient information previously.)

» Have a basic understanding of the person's situation and begin to build trust with them.

» Assessors need to be professional, honest, open and approachable.

» Assessors should listen, repeat or paraphrase facts to ensure that they have an accurate understanding of what is going on and have made notes, if appropriate.

» Recognise that the person being assessed is a part of 'something' ie use a holistic/whole-person approach.

» Know what is going on and available in the wider community and how that individual might contribute or 'fit' within that.

» People want whoever is carrying out the assessment to remember that they have a past and that you are just seeing a snapshot in time of their life. Assessors should attempt to see the wider picture.

» Assessments should focus on outcomes and explain what the possible outcomes might be.

» Assessors need to be realistic, and make it clear that they can't fix everything in one session and that this is an ongoing process.

» Likewise, people being assessed seek clarity. It is important to be clear about who is making any given decision. If the findings of an assessment need to be put forward to a manager before any decision is made, this needs to be made clear from the start. Similarly, people need to know that they have a right to appeal against the outcome of an assessment.

» People being assessed prefer professionals to be friendly and approachable, but to remember that they are not a friend.

» Don't use jargon.

## Practical **task**

Think about a service you have been involved in providing for someone (not even necessarily in relation to health and social care). Try and *honestly* rate your own contribution to the above ideals from a score of 1 (needs more work) to 5 (excellent).

## Personal **reflection**

While avoiding jargon seems so obvious, we all become 'professionalised' into our own ways of working and the shortcuts we make in our conversations. I was recently speaking to my sister about a relative of ours, who was being assisted by the local authority to change accommodation. When asked by my sister for an update I answered straightaway:

*They are waiting to identify an appropriate property for her.*

*To which she replied: What, find her a house?*

## Practical **task**

### Where to start – what to say?

While every assessment of a carer is different, and I would by no means want to put words into people's mouths, in some situations inexperienced assessors may find that they 'dry up' at important moments. While some authorities have a check list of questions to run through, for others the assessment is reliant on the assessor's professional judgement (Milner, Myers and O'Byrne, 2015) and mode and models of inquiry. Working off a basic script can sometimes be helpful. If this is a scenario you have encountered, try to consider asking open questions that might cover the following:

» What are the issues that lead you to get in touch?

» Who is being affected by the situation? How, when and where? Who is involved?

» Tell me about a 'typical' day. What does/would help/hinder?

» Tell me about your idea of a 'perfect' day.

» What are the strengths in your caring relationship, and how may they be built on?

» What factors are present in the background (eg employment, divorce, illness)?

» What are your worst fears?

One of the key elements to remember when considering assessments is to be aware that any assessment has a power dimension, which will shape and determine the relationship (Brammer and Boylan, 2017). Practitioners need to understand the unique circumstances of individuals and approach any assessment critically and analytically being aware of the wider structural factors that impinge on the lives of family carers and those in receipt of care.

This chapter has considered issues relating to the notion of professionals and professionalism, and the ways in which carers are sometimes viewed by professionals: as a resource, a co-worker, a co-client, a professional or an expert. In addition, we have been exploring some pertinent issues relating to carers' needs assessments under the Care Act (2014a), taking account of these factors in terms of their likely influence.

Discussing the requirements needed to complete an assessment, this chapter has offered practical examples as well as personal reflections.

In the following chapter we turn our attention to issues relating to research and practice and how research may support the work of practitioners with family carers.

## Taking it further

1. This useful guide is helpful for those practitioners looking to start or develop working together initiatives. https://camera-pupsmd.org.uk/pdf/working-together-guide.pdf

2. For a useful and interesting discussion regarding a diverse and inclusive approach to assessment see Chapter 8. *Shedding Light on the Expert Witness Role in Child Welfare Work*, by Trish Walsh in Witkin, S (ed) (2011) *Social Construction and Social Work Practice: Interpretations and Innovations*. Columbia University Press.

# References

Brammer, A and Boylan, J (eds) (2017) *Critical Issues in Social Work Law.* London: Palgrave Macmillan.

Brodaty, H and Donkin, M (2009) Family caregivers of people with dementia. *Dialogues in Clinical Neuroscience, 11*(2): 217–28.

Carers UK (2015) *Valuing Carers 2015 – The Rising Value of Carers' Support.* University of Sheffield, University of Leeds and CIRCLE, published by Carers UK.

Chapman, A (2015) Using the assessment process to overcome Imposter Syndrome in mature students. *Journal of Further and Higher Education, 41*(2): 112–19.

Department of Health (DH) (2014) Care Act 2014 Fact Sheet 4: Personalising Care and Support Planning. Department of Health: London.

Feldon, P (2017) *The Social Worker's Guide to the Care Act 2014.* St Albans: Critical Publishing.

Flexner, A (2001). Is social work a profession? *Research on Social Work Practice, 11*(2): 152–65.

Hammick, M, Freeth, D, Koppel, I, Reeves, S and Barr, H (2007) A best evidence systematic review of interprofessional education: BEME Guide no. 9. *Medical Teacher, 29*(8): 735–51.

Manthorpe, J, Iliffe, S and Eden, A (2003) Testing Twigg and Atkin's typology of caring: a study of primary care professionals' perceptions of dementia care using a modified focus group method. *Health & Social Care in the Community, 11*(6): 477–85.

Milner, J, Myers, S and O'Byrne, P (2015) *Assessment in Social Work.* Palgrave Macmillan.

Ramsey, E and Brown, D (2017) Feeling like a fraud: helping students renegotiate their academic identities. *College & Undergraduate Libraries, 25*(1): 86–90.

Rollero, C (2016) The experience of men caring for a partner with multiple sclerosis. *Journal of Nursing Scholarship, 48*(5): 482–9.

Roos, S (2002) *Chronic Sorrow: A Living Loss.* New York: Brunner-Routledge.

Schwehr B (2014) How the Care Act 2014 will shape assessment and support planning – a legal opinion. www.communitycare.co.uk/2014/02/27/care-act-2014-will-shape-assessment-support-planning-legal-opinion/ [accessed 1 April 2018].

SCIE (2009) Interprofessional and inter-agency collaboration (IPIAC). www.scie.org.uk/publications/elearning/ipiac/ [accessed 1 April 2018].

SCIE (2014) The Care Act: assessment and eligibility. www.scie.org.uk/care-act-2014/assessment-and-eligibility/ [accessed 1 April 2018].

Twigg, J and Atkin, K (1994) *Carers Perceived: Policy and Practice in Informal Care.* Buckingham: Open University Press.

UK Government (2014a) Care Act 2014. www.legislation.gov.uk/ukpga/2014/23/contents/enacted [accessed 1 April 2018].

UK Government (2014b) The Care and Support (Eligibility Criteria) Regulations 2014. www.legislation.gov.ukwww.legislation.gov.uk/ukdsi/2014/9780111124185 [accessed 1 April 2018].

UK Government (2014c) Using the Care Act guidance. www.gov.uk/government/publications/care-actstatutory-guidance/ care-and-support-statutory-guidance [accessed 1 April 2018].

Walsh, T (2011) Shedding Light on the Expert Witness Role in Child Welfare Work. In *Social Construction and Social Work Practice: Interpretations and Innovations.* New York: Columbia University Press.

Yesufu-Udechuku, A, Harrison, B, Mayo-Wilson, E, Young, N, Woodhams, P, Shiers, D, Kuipers, E and Kendall, T (2015) Interventions to improve the experience of caring for people with severe mental illness: systematic review and meta-analysis. *The British Journal of Psychiatry*, 206(4): 268–74.

# Chapter 6 | Research and practice

Continuing the discussions started in Chapter 2, this chapter looks at research, what it is and what it might tell us in general terms, as well as what research may offer our practice as practitioners. Looking at what the research says about some of the effects of care-giving, including the impact and experiences of care-giving in various settings and with different groups, this chapter explores the relationship between research and practice with carers. The 'ethics of care' debate (Gilligan, 1982; Kittay and Myers, 1987; Mayeroff, 1971) and debates around ethical reasoning will be noted. Although as noted in Chapter 3, research indicates that carers are not a homogenous group; it has been suggested that the tendency is to research only the most prominent groups in any category, and those carers from a Black and ethnic minority background, or carers who may not fit into a specific 'box', may find there is little in the literature that represents their own experiences.

As a starting point, it is worth unpicking exactly what we mean by 'research' before we go on to explore what the research might tell us about care and the effects of care-giving. The word 'research' is derived from the French word 'chercher' – a verb meaning to look for. Research involves (re)-looking for new knowledge and understanding about a given topic. For a more formal definition, the UK policy framework for health and social care (www.hra.nhs.uk/.../1068/uk-policy-framework-health-social-care-research.pdf) research states that research is defined as an attempt to derive generalisable or transferable new knowledge to answer or refine relevant questions with scientifically sound methods.

So, it is about looking for and (hopefully) finding knowledge to help solve problems, or to extend our understanding of an area. The UK policy framework sees research as being a core function of health and well-being and fundamental to developing and extending our understanding.

Therefore, it would follow that in order to develop our understanding of some of the issues and challenges facing carers, as well as being able to work competently and confidently with carers, research is essential. Keeping up to date about practice issues and new evidence that may come to light is important in order to be a well-rounded professional. Understanding what works, why, where, how and when are areas that are important for practitioners in all fields.

The ways in which knowledge is 'looked for' varies according to its philosophical underpinnings. Research methodology refers to these underpinnings of research – the 'why' you are doing research in a particular way. Research methods are the 'nuts and bolts' of *how* you do the research. For example, a semi-structured research interview is a method, a way of carrying out research.

Research has a language of its own and it may appear incomprehensible the first time one encounters it. Words such as 'epistemology', 'ontology', 'empiricism', 'interpretivism' and 'constructivism' may be overwhelming for the first-time practitioner researcher; however, with time and experience comes familiarity. If you have to undertake research as part of your course of study, or for your practice, then do try not to be overwhelmed; make a glossary of terms that you may encounter to refer to – and remember, research is as much, if not more, about those practical attributes of actually 'doing' and reading, as it is about the terminology applied.

The history of research in health and social care is closely linked with philosophical theories that inform two main methodological paradigms, or 'ways of seeing' the world (Berger, 1972). These can be represented (broadly) as being either positivistic or interpretivist (Hughes and Sharrock, 1997) and both make claims regarding the nature of reality, our understanding of the nature of truth and what may or may not be regarded as knowledge (Hothersall, 2016; Howell, 2013). These two (broad) categorisations can also be described as representing the quantitative and the qualitative traditions – the former having its emphasis on the use of numbers, the latter on the use of narratives as ways of seeing and describing the world. With a quantitative approach to research and inquiry, the aim is to test (objectively) a particular hypothesis, and the researcher is more likely to describe an issue and explain a phenomenon by using measurable data, such as numbers and surveys, which are then analysed using statistical and mathematical data, with the results presented in the form of charts and tables. A qualitative approach to research is seen as more subjectively oriented, providing insights into phenomena as well as *developing* hypotheses. Its methods include interviews and focus groups, and these are used to try to find answers for why and how people behave, think and feel.

However, this rather simplistic dualism does little to portray accurately the most effective ways of inquiring into the nature of reality, as both have their inherent strengths and weaknesses. As such, a third paradigm must be referred to – one that attempts (quite successfully) to 'bridge' what for some might seem like a methodological 'chasm' – mixed-methods research (MMR). In this, methods representative of either approach can be utilised to inquire/research, with the only prescription being to use the method(s) that work best for a given research problem.

Put simply, research inquiry is more than a set of skills; it is a way of looking at and thinking about the world, and a way of asking questions and seeking explanations and understanding and gaining insight, underpinned of course by being critically engaged with the available research in your particular domain of practice.

See 'Taking it further' at the end of this chapter for ideas for finding out more about the different ways of approaching research in health and social care.

It has been noted (ironically within academic scholarly research) that social workers rarely, or never, read scholarly research (Jeffrey, 2013) and I imagine similar comments may be made about many other health and social care practitioners, yet it is research and the associated findings that guide and shape much of what we do every day in society. Well-informed research leads to well-informed and thoughtful practice, but only if opportunities exist for it to be read, observed and developed. More time needs to be spent on identifying how busy practitioners, including social workers, can be supported to stay up to date.

For health and social care practitioners to do what they need to do, in order to provide a useful and necessary service, they need to base their interventions on evidence. Who, or what that evidence is based upon is debatable, and open to critique, but actions need to be based on something that might be rationalised – even if it is 'instinct'. How do practitioners know what they need to know in order to do what they need to do? (Hothersall, 2016). While practice wisdom, instinct and intuition have a lot to offer, few of us would want our GP to practise by instinct alone; rather we would prefer that they draw on a body of knowledge informed by past experiences and indicators of success. In a similar way, if a social worker is removing a child from their birth family to be placed in the care of the local authority, this action needs to be based upon research. We need to know, for example, what the research tells us about children whose parents use illegal substances and who may have a recorded history of violence and abuse, and then both be able to make a judgement based on the facts as they are presented to us, but also to be able to draw on a body of knowledge that tells us, in the example given above, that children are more at risk of neglect and abuse if they remain in the situation with parents who are abusive and are drug users. Therefore, one of the functions of research in health and social care practice is to support practitioners to find out what may be possible solutions to problems and also potential ways of mitigating such dilemmas.

## Reflective **task**

Think about the word 'inquiry' as opposed to 'research' and then consider the last time you inquired about something. What did you do and what did you find out? Where did this come from and can you remember what it was?

Now begin to consider where you might go to see if there is any academic or work-related inquiry or research information about a topic you are interested in.

When considering the task, you may have said that the last inquiry you carried out was for something personal – not work related. Perhaps you are thinking of booking a holiday? You would no doubt have 'researched' the topic, asked questions of other people, looked at websites and brochures as well as reading accounts from other visitors or holiday makers. Chances are when answering the exercise above you said you looked to social media as the first source of news on a given topic.

The 2017 Reuters Institute Digital News Report (www.digitalnewsreport.org/survey/2017/overview-key-findings-2017) found that there were different market-based preferences for how people discover and access news, with people in the UK being more likely to go directly to a website or app. Facebook, Youtube and Whats App were seen as the top social networks for news. Online print from 'traditional' news sources is still seen as the first point of call for those 'harder' stories, whereas newer social media platforms are explored for 'softer' issues. There is also an age difference in how news is received, with younger people more likely to use social media as opposed to print. So how then do health and social care practitioners find out what they need to know? For some practitioners, the use of algorithms to choose news stories and key issues in research and practice may be preferred, as they suggest it removes editorial preference and may provide a counterbalance to 'fake' news. In practice, however, there seems to be a gap between what research tells us, and how and where it is produced, and most importantly, how it is applied – if indeed it is applied – in practice.

Practitioners need to be able to read and refer to research in order to provide a credible evidence base to the work they do. Being 'research-minded' is in essence being curious about the world in which we live, and being able to then apply that curiosity towards your work. Using research may help to offer a wider perspective on any given situation; it allows you to make better decisions based on evidence. Additionally, by reading research your knowledge and understanding of a given topic will increase.

Inquiry, or research by practitioners and more so carried out by carers and the person in receipt of care, is still infrequent; and yet who best to inform and advise on a particular process or intervention than those on whom it has most direct impact? Research within practice is used to evaluate as well as develop a knowledge base to further enhance information, and in the situation regarding work with carers and with those in receipt of care, it is an essential component. Practitioner-led research may support professionals to challenge assumptions (their own and others') as well as maintain their enthusiasm and professional curiosity.

The internet is a fabulous source of research information; however, it can be overwhelming in the amount of detail available at the touch of a key. Remember, though, even in the twenty-first century it is not always the first (and only) way to obtain information.

## Case example

Phoebe and Everleigh are health and social care undergraduates and have been given a class project to find out about services that are available for carers in their local area. Their tutor has insisted that students do not use the internet, but instead go out and find out for themselves.

Initially, the students were completely stumped and did not know where to begin. After a brief moan about the tutor, who they decided was a dinosaur, the students decided to visit the local library in the centre of town. From there they found information about a variety of services and collected some leaflets. One was to do with a coffee morning for carers to attend while their relatives with dementia attended a memory support session. Phoebe and Everleigh decided that they would give it a go – tempted by the prospect of free coffee, if nothing else – and they thought they would quite like to speak to carers. When they did, they found that by speaking to carers over coffee they had a much clearer idea of services that were available, and recognised that they would otherwise not have known about these services. Additionally, both students felt that they gained from meeting people directly. Some of the stories they heard, and the examples of care-giving situations, challenges and rewards, have stayed with them for much longer than just reading about caring on a web page.

When they returned to university with the information they had gathered, they felt better able to deliver a presentation about services for carers, and spoke passionately about the need for support for carers in their

> local community. Other students who admitted 'cheating' and using their phones to find out information began to feel that they had missed out, and later in the module were less able to recall the relevant information.
>
> Communicating at a human level makes the reality of people's lives much more focused, is more memorable and affects a response in a way that reading or researching on the internet does not.

As you will see then, using the internet is not without its pitfalls. Where, then, does this leave health and social care practitioners who want to inquire, to explore and to expand their understanding of a particular topic? Not everyone has the time, resources or contacts to be able to meet people face to face, as in the example above.

Topics that attract research interest (and funding) may go through phases of popularity or media attention. This may be dependent on a variety of factors; for example, developments in legislation, celebrity endorsement and media attention – and how some topics attract a lot of media attention, and others less so on any given topic – is beyond the remit of this book to consider. Suffice to say that it appears that issues related to carers and caring are generally low on the list of priorities for media attention and research funding.

The Economic and Social Research Council (ESRC) is the UK's largest organisation for funding research on economic and social issues. It funds research across a variety of topics and arranges research activities into social science topics including 'health and well-being' and 'society'. With a total budget of approximately £202 million for 2017/ 18 the ESRC supports independent and high quality research.

The priorities for the ESRC (2016–20) are:

- » climate change;
- » innovation in health and social care;
- » trust and global governance in a turbulent age;
- » mental health;
- » housing;
- » productivity;
- » understanding the macroeconomy.

Clearly, research relating to care-giving may be incorporated into most, if not all, of the topics above in some shape or form; for example, in the research priority that is innovation in health and social care, there is an emphasis on working with people with dementia as a case study. In the priority that is mental health the influence of relationships is noted. In essence, one could draw out several key areas relating to care and care-giving across a variety of areas, some more explicitly than others. How the findings and recommendations from such research are produced and translated into accessible formats that are read by practitioners themselves, and by carers is a complex issue. Ring-fenced study time for practitioners may be one answer, perhaps identifying and exploring ways in which they might translate the findings from research recommendations into their own practice. The adage of 'be a lifelong learner' is relevant and timely, and yet one which may be seen as a luxury by many organisations.

# Student dissertations

Many health and social care students now have to incorporate some aspect of research into their studies at both undergraduate and postgraduate level. Often giving students an opportunity to explore in greater depth an area or subject of particular interest for those programmes of study that incorporate a practice placement, a research dissertation is an excellent chance to investigate a specific topic that may have relevance and practical use. Undertaking a research project enables students to develop their research skills and knowledge while at the same time may generate new and important research findings for practice (Campbell et al, 2017).

Student dissertations generally follow a similar format:

» formulate a question or area that needs investigating;

» review the literature on the topic;

» independent research;

» justification of the methodology, methods and analysis;

» present and discuss findings (Carey, 2013).

## Reflective **task**

Key areas to consider:

How might you demonstrate your 'professional or academic curiosity'?

How might exploring this area benefit the areas (individuals or groups) under study?

How might 'doing' research help to develop your own knowledge and understanding?

How will you disseminate the findings of your research?

# Social media

Just as research methods have become more sophisticated and taken account of technological advances, for example, the sophisticated software to search literature and analyse data, as well as the growth in research methods such as photovoice and videographics, so too has the rise in social media as a tool for professionals working with carers.

Developing an online presence in a professional sense may be problematic for health and social care practitioners. The approach to social media from employers has, in some instances, been slow to materialise and cautious. Additionally, recommendations and guidance on the use of social media are unlikely to keep pace with advancing technology. There is a possibility of practitioners being unsure of their boundaries and becoming anxious regarding their own use of social media in a professional capacity, and of the message their own digital footprint sends out about them. Recommendations following a serious case review into the murder of a child by its mother's partner, from the Wolverhampton Safeguarding Childrens Board (5 January 2018) www.wolverhamptonsafeguarding.org.uk/safeguarding-children-and-young-people/i-work-with-children-young-people-families/serious-case-reviews-and-other-learning-reviews/serious-case-review-child-g, included the need to consider how best to enable practitioners to access relevant public-facing social media to enhance their assessments. Exploring information that is in the public domain via social media may inform and support triangulation of information and add to the quality of assessments by health and social care practitioners. However, this is an extremely complex area and obtaining and using information in this way needs to be considered sensitively and in accordance with one's own agency policies and protocols. Recent literature supports this view and suggests that organisations need to ensure that they have up-to-date policies to define social media use and misuse (Sage and Sage, 2016).

If we take 'social media' to be the swift development of the use of apparatus of technology by people in order to interact, communicate, learn and participate in society (Caplan and Purser, 2017), then it is relatively easy to identify potential ethical, professional, practical and confidentiality issues. Taking the use of Facebook alone, the digital footprint one produces may result in a vast amount of information which employers, colleagues, clients and customers are able to access at the touch of a button. Organisations such as the British Association of Social Workers (BASW) advise against accepting requests from carers and service users as online friends in a personal network, recognising the pitfalls, including the potential for coercion and potential litigation.

The sensitivity of the situation of working with service users and carers, coupled with the benefits of providing a service at a greatly reduced cost, is a dilemma many organisations are wrestling with. While few local authority social service departments may have a Twitter account per se, the people that lead such departments do, as do those in positions of power – for example, the chief social worker for adults and the chief social worker for children (Lyn Romeo and Isabelle Trowler, at time of writing) – are active in their use of social media to disseminate information. Communicating online offers many benefits and is significantly less costly than attending a meeting or a conference. Of course, issues of data protection, confidentiality and anonymity need to be considered; they are important factors, and should be part of a professional's training. Given the rapid growth of technology, such training needs to be an ongoing activity in order for practitioners to keep up to date. Likewise, many health and social care practitioners may need to be equipped with digital skills to be able to access information as well as ensuring their contribution is ethical. As a way of communicating with service users and carers, digital media is surely a growth area. Digital literacy is a much needed skill for health and social care practitioners in the twenty-first century and if this is to include incorporating the outward-facing use of social media by service users and carers with whom you are working, clear guidance needs to be provided by employers.

## Practical **task**

Find out what the guidelines are from your organisation, or university, regarding use of digital and social media. How easy are they to access? Would you be able to use a carer's 'outward-facing' social media account perhaps as collateral in an assessment? See if you can find out how frequently guidelines are updated and by whom.

Research specifically to do with care and the effects of care-giving is wide and covers a broad spectrum of typologies of care. The characteristic of the carer (for example, older carer, spousal carer, sibling carer, young carer) and/or the diagnosis of the person in receipt (for example, adult with learning difficulties, older person with dementia, child with autism) of care appear to be predominant themes within carers' research literature.

More general research to do with carers and the person in receipt of care includes those questions asked more generally, for example, through surveys. These provide an extremely useful way of identifying problems and correlations. For example:

» What percentage of the population in a given area, over the age of 65 has dementia?

» How many children of primary school age have been the subject of a referral to CAMHS?

Many research projects and associated findings regarding carers tend to be drawn from small-scale qualitative projects utilising relatively small samples of carers. For example, when exploring the experiences of older carers of adults with learning disabilities, Cairns et al's 2013 study involved interviewing only six mothers and two fathers of adults with learning difficulties to obtain an understanding of their experiences and views of care of their sons or daughters in the future. Likewise, Dillenburger and McKerr's 2011 study involved 29 older parent-carers who were interviewed to explore their perspectives on long-term care arrangements.

The small scale of such projects, while valuable for producing a richness and depth of data that may otherwise have been missed, needs to be balanced with longitudinal projects and those with a high number of respondents. All research involves time and effort on behalf of the researcher, but also on behalf of the particpants. It has been suggested by Mockford, in relation to carers and hospital discharge for people with dementia, that 'Carers who may feel their world is far removed from the academic world may not ordinarily participate in research studies' (Mockford, 2015: 21). However, research that involves people who use services and are controlled by them seems to be gaining momentum, according to Beresford (2012). In the context of developing a more focused and sustainable model of research, different ways of supporting carers, people in receipt of care and practitioners as researchers are needed. We might ask – who better to identify topics worthy of research attention than those people immersed in that topic? Academics may be criticised for failing to keep in touch with the real world; however, as we know, caring is likely to touch the majority of people at some point in their lives, and bring the 'real world' into sharp focus for many.

Universities, like many other public institutions, need to make a more sustainable investment in communities that goes beyond tokenism and which enables practitioners to develop, nurture and contribute to research with those for whom it has greatest impact. Practitioners who carry out research may be able to offer a challenge and/or critique of current work and develop the emancipatory potential of health and social care practice (Hardwick and Worsley, 2010). Practice-based research is still a relatively underdeveloped area, and imperatives within the Knowledge and Skills Statements for Social Workers highlight the need to address these shortcomings.

# Ethical debates in relation to care

As an approach to understanding care and care-giving particularly when linked with issues of morality, there are many ethical considerations that arise. Dilemmas occur every day: issues to do with human rights and freedoms; the longstanding gender stereotypes that exist which see women as having caring natures; the role of society and the impact of race, ethnicity and gender are some examples of general ethical dilemmas. On a personal level consider the following.

» Do you give money to a homeless person or buy yourself a cup of coffee on the way to work?

» Do you help your elderly neighbour carry their shopping into their house even though it means you will miss your bus?

» Do you tell your best friend you have seen her partner embracing another woman?

Ways of dealing with such ethical dilemmas and arriving at a reasonable outcome for all those concerned is complex. How people choose to approach and address such dilemmas varies, and some theorists believe that there is a difference in how women and men deal with ethical issues relating to care in particular and how this then influences decisions about provision and supply of care.

The ethic of the care debate focuses on the ethical theory that puts care and relationships at the centre of any moral action. Care, concern and responsibility towards others, along with a connection with people, are seen as key factors to understanding an ethical approach to care.

Everyone has personal values and characteristics that guide and shape everyday actions, particularly when faced with a dilemma or when a decision is to be made. Ethical reasoning is the ability to assess and identify a given course of action. In professional as well as in personal life ethical dilemmas occur every day. Our behaviour has consequences for ourselves and for the welfare of others, and how we approach and deal with this relates to our reasoning.

Early debates around the ethics of care debate have their roots in the work of Carol Gilligan in the 1980s. For Gilligan (1982), women use different ethical reasoning – ie an 'ethics of care' approach to life – whereas men use an ethics of justice to inform their daily lives. Put simply, the ethics of care approach can be seen as an approach to care that is based on responsibilities and relationships whereas an ethics of justice approach is based on rights and rules (Tronto, 1993). It is important to note, of course, that the first of these approaches is not exclusively the province of women, and such a point has been a critique of the often linear demarcation between debates to do with care and justice ethics.

Feminist writers were among the first to debate and develop research on care and highlight and dispute what was seen as a 'natural' female activity. Feminists call for the discourse of rights and justice to be substituted for the discourse of care and believe that the notion of care itself as it is seen in its current form needs to be unpicked and dismantled. Care ethics originally developed as an alternative to the moral theories of Kantian deontology (duty) and Utilitarian consequentialism (the end justifies the means). The ethics of care as a discourse has been widely debated; for example, can one truly care if one is forced to so do by psychological, financial or emotional imperative?

Later writers call for an approach that incorporates both these ideas – the notions of both justice *and* care in order to facilitate new understandings on the social concept and context of care. It is beyond the remit of this book to discuss and debate this philosophical perspective in any depth; however, for practitioners working with family carers a basic awareness of some of the debates and discussions that exist may be key to developing their own understanding of the slippery notion that is care, and of recognising the importance of ethics and ethical reasoning within that.

In terms of justifying or critiquing the place of carers, the ethics of care debate may be useful for practitioners and students to explore in greater depth.

# Caring as a positive experience

For many carers, the notion of care as a 'burden' as noted by many commentators (Papastavrou et al, 2007; Pinquart and Sörensen, 2003) does not equate with their own day-to-day experiences. Assessments and the perspectives practitioners may hold might focus on a deficit model of caring, ie what providing care to another person has taken away from the carer's life, not what it has added. Reports of depression (Loi et al, 2016; Emerson et al, 2010), physical health problems (Miravitlles et al, 2015; Carers UK, 2012), poverty (Aldridge and Hughes, 2016; Keating et al, 2014) and stress (Fox et al, 2010; Stoltz et al, 2004) are frequently found in the literature concerning carers.

It is important to acknowledge that there is another side to this, and increasingly research studies can be identified that report a positive aspect to the provision of care; for example, Ribeiro and Paul's 2008 study of older men providing care for their wives reported 'satisfaction' and 'perceived social honour' as being attached to the role. Other studies (Li and Loke, 2013) reported carers as developing an enhanced relationship with the care-receiver, obtaining a feeling of being rewarded, as well as a sense of personal growth, and a perception of personal satisfaction. Carers may see their role as giving meaning and purpose to their lives and as ways of developing emotional skills such as patience, tenacity and compassion, as well as practical skills such as budgeting, coordinating meetings, time-keeping, to say nothing of those skills loosely grouped under the term 'personal care'. Being able to bathe or shower someone and still allow them to retain their dignity is a skill not to be underestimated. Being a carer therefore may well facilitate the enhancement and growth of one's own personal development.

Some research literature offers a discussion of positive aspects that caring brings about – see, for example, McCann et al (2015), who note the greater bonds developed between carer and care recipient, and carer's satisfaction at seeing the person they are caring for appreciate the care provided. These positive features of caring are disproportionately recorded when exploring challenges associated with the caring role. There is an imbalance and the general emphasis of research accounts does focus on the notion of care-giving as a burden.

# Resilience

The concept of 'resilience' has been seen in recent years as an important one for practitioners to assimilate and demonstrate in their practice. For example, in January 2017 the Health and Care Professions Council (HCPC) introduced a new standard of proficiency for social workers to incorporate resilience. The standards of proficiency are designed to set out what a social worker in England needs to know, once qualified, in order to apply to be registered with the HCPC – for more details go to www.hpc-uk.org/assets/documents/10003B08Standardsofproficiency-SocialworkersinEngland.pdf.

Regarding resilience, the guidelines state that a social worker needs to be able to identify and apply strategies to build professional resilience. To this I would add that carers need also to be able to apply strategies to develop their own resilience, and that health and social care practitioners need to look at ways of developing their *personal* resilience also.

So what do we mean by resilience? How might health and social care practitioners and carers begin to identify and apply strategies to build such resilience?

Likewise, how might people working with carers be able to support them to develop and draw on their own resilience? Life can be extremely difficult at times; a catastrophic fire, a terrorist attack, a flood, the death of a loved one, and being made redundant, are all examples of some of the severe challenges life brings about for people. Following the immediate reactions of shock, horror, anger and disbelief, many people then seem to adapt and to find ways of dealing with these feelings and not go under. Likewise, for practitioners working with people experiencing life-changing events, how too might they adapt and build on their own practice to develop a 'professional' resilience?

## Reflective **task**

Think about a time you have experienced sadness, conflict or adversity. Try and identify what helped you at that time, perhaps a comment made, or a kind gesture from a friend. Reflect on how you may draw on that experience to develop your practice and/or personal situation.

Brian was an only child who had an extremely close relationship with his mother. His father was in the navy and spent many years living overseas. Brian's widowed mother died when she was 84 and he was 50 – not an especially uncommon situation for people of their age.

The first time Brian went shopping after the funeral he would look at other people of similar age to his Mum in the shops and think about the fact that those people must have had similar devastating losses at some point in their lives. He said he wondered how they survived this awful emotional and at times raw physical pain that threatened to engulf him. How do people find the strength to carry on? He saw people much older than himself walking around, getting on with their day-to-day lives, and yet the rational part of him acknowledged that to have reached that age, they too must have been through some extremely challenging and painful times. Brian wondered how people seem to manage to function 'normally' even though they themselves must have experienced great sadness, conflict and adversity at times.

How do some people manage to deal with some very difficult situations? Resilience is the word used to describe such a concept, being seen as the ability to recover from difficulties or to bounce back, like a rubber ball thrown against a wall, from experiences or situations which are challenging. Resilience is a necessary component for a successful life, and the resilient carer is one who adapts and accepts what they cannot change. Resilience is seen as an 'ordinary' not an 'extraordinary' characteristic; rather it is a way of accepting and recognising that life is unpredictable; it is never going to be a bed of roses, and it is about being tolerant about what comes along. People's personalities, backgrounds, resources and the ways they cope with challenges are seen as key to developing resilience. Resilience and vulnerability might both be seen as internal characteristics; these are shaped by a complex web of factors, including 'nature' and 'nurture' as well as how individuals perceive and respond to situations.

What resources might professionals draw on to develop their own resilience?

Do they differ? If, as stated in Chapter 1, many of us will be carers at some point in our life-course, the likelihood is that the lines will be blurred. Many professionals will undertake personal caring roles for friends and relatives and many carers may be in professional roles. It is difficult at times to separate those professional and personal characteristics that help to identify and apply strategies of resilience. However you approach the topic, in essence it is such areas as community, family relations, social support, social cohesion and participation that have an influence on the likelihood of achieving successful resilience. According to research, other characteristics which have a bearing on successful resilience include gender, age, ethnicity, health status, the neighbourhood in which you live or work, as well as one's involvement with health and social care and employment (Windle and Bennett, 2012). Whichever way you choose to look at it, resilience is never just down to an individual factor, rather, it appears to be a complex interaction between personal 'internal' characteristics and those external factors that are outside of our control.

It is important to recognise too that people might be resilient to some situations, but not to others, and on some occasions and not others – it is contextual.

Looking at literature on resilience, commentators suggest that there are three main areas that are seen as the foundation on which resilience is built. These are discussed specifically in relation to children, but have, I believe, wider application.

These are described as being:

> » a secure base, bringing about a sense of belonging and security;

> » good self-esteem, in essence an internal sense of worth and competence;

> » a sense of self-efficacy; this is taken to refer to a sense of control of one's own situation, along with a realistic understanding of one's own personal strengths and limitations (Gilligan, 1997).

## Practical **task**

Taking note of the case study regarding Rob and Sylvia in Chapter 4:

Jot down your thoughts about factors that may (a) minimise (hinder) and (b) maximise (nurture), Sylvia's resilience.

In answering the above you may have included for (a) such factors as her vulnerability and the adversity she faces when attempting to deal with services designed to support Rob, the uncertainty his condition brings about and management of his unpredictable emotional state; for (b) such factors as Sylvia's tenacity in developing her own interests, her sense of humour as well as her strong sense of duty.

Factors that may help to develop and sustain a carer's resilience include having a positive outlook on life. While this may seem 'Pollyannaish,' having someone else around to talk to and let off steam is also a helpful factor in developing resilience. Good health, adequate financial income and a safe and secure place to live also play a part in determining the level of resilience, as well as having some practical and domestic help around the home (Windle and Bennett, 2012). For others (McCann et al, 2015) carer resilience is developed by carers seeing their role as satisfying and as providing a purpose to their own lives. Therefore, by drawing on support from others and maintaining their own well-being, carers may find their own resilience deepens.

When it comes to interactions with professionals, for carers their resilience is more likely to be strengthened, unsurprisingly, by empathic support that pays attention to strengths and achievements. Carers may also benefit from regular activities and a social structure that is supportive of them. A key factor in developing and sustaining successful resilience for many carers is having sympathetic friends who accept the situation for what it is, and having supportive wider family members who offer help without being asked. For some carers, knowing different 'practical' ways of coping – for example, using mindfulness techniques, meditation or 'tapping', and being sufficiently confident to apply them when needed could be helpful. Additionally, to be able to use the ability to separate oneself either psychologically or physically from a stressful situation may also be a key to developing and maintaining a caring relationship and not 'going under' when it gets tough. How carers navigate and negotiate their own well-being depends a lot on their state of resilience, or ability to 'bounce back' from problematic situations.

Practitioners have a role to play in assessing the needs of carers and supporting carers in their role. This may sound simplistic, however, it is a key factor that should not be underestimated. Adequate and empathic support through an assessment – now seen as an intervention in itself under the Care Act (2014) – may be the difference between carers 'going on' and carers 'going under'.

## Case example

Lita was a carer for her sister (Jana) who had severe learning difficulties, and following the death of their mother Jana moved into Lita's flat. Over time the two sisters developed their own routines and ways of dealing with life together. Lita says it was not the retirement she had envisaged for herself, but that she was making the best of the situation, and adapting to the changes and challenges associated with caring for her sister. Throughout her career as a medical receptionist, Lita prided herself on her assertiveness and her ability to solve problems. She believed that she was extremely self-aware, and that all of these qualities helped to maintain her resilience when the situation with Jana became problematic due to Jana's increasing anxiety.

One day Jana was admitted to hospital having suffered a CVA (stroke). She remained in hospital for several weeks. During this time, despite having more time to herself and the opportunity to catch up with her sleep, meet friends and take up her hobbies once more, Lita became increasingly low in mood. The uncertainty of the situation, coupled as it was with worries about her sister's health and longevity had, as she put it, 'severely dented her optimism and positive attitude to life'. In other words, her ability to be resilient through one set of circumstances did not necessarily translate to another. As adversities cumulate, the ability to 'bounce back' lessens and sometimes it is the smallest thing that can finally be too much. It is important to note that while developing and building resilience may be the key to a long and successful career, it is not a substitute for the root cause of many problems that affect one's resilience. For practitioners these may be matters such as high case loads, and demanding clients, whereas for carers the root cause may be lack of sleep, and isolation.

In any discussions regarding resilience it is important to note that by emphasising the importance of individual resilience, whether from a professional or a personal perspective, in no way do I wish to undermine the impact of the wider environment and what may be the root causes: nor do I wish to understate the importance of recognising and tackling such causes at source.

Take a moment to consider the above points in relation to carers and what you know about carers thus far. Think about ways in which an understanding of carer resilience might be identified during an assessment, and also of ways of embedding resilience into the assessment process. What do you think is the reality for carers' resilience considering:

we know many carers are likely to be isolated?

we know many carers are in poor health?

we know many carers struggle financially?

we know many carers are unemployed?

# Professionals' resilience

Just as a myriad of factors influence and shape the likelihood of successful carer resilience, so too do a number of varied and fluctuating factors influence the likelihood of health and social care practitioners developing a successful 'professional' resilience. The resilience of practitioners is more likely to be shaped by the culture in which you practise and includes having a positive outlook, feeling you have supportive colleagues and having clear goals and aspirations to work towards. For many professionals the key to successful resilience and a long-term career is the ability to maintain a balance between independence and dependence on others, so, for example, knowing when to act autonomously and when to seek help. For practitioners, having the presence of a positive supervisor or a mentor, as well as having role models who show and share the 'practice wisdom' needed for a long-term career, is also fundamental.

Key to professional resilience is also having a feeling of control over one's destiny and having opportunities for suitable work that both stretches and is appropriately challenging.

There is a high turnover of staff associated with many of the caring professions; for example, in adult social care there is an overall turnover rate of 25.4 per cent. This equates to approximately 300,000 workers leaving their roles each year (Skills for Care, 2015). Similarly, a recently published analysis of the Nursing and Midwifery Council (NMC) register indicated that the number of nurses leaving the profession is greater than the number joining (NMC, 2017). Reasons cited for people leaving include feeling undervalued at work and excessive job demands, as well as low pay and poor working conditions. Working within health and social care settings may be stressful; you will be working with people who may be vulnerable, unpredictable and unwell. Clearly, there is a need for a healthy work-life balance in order to maintain a long successful and hopefully enjoyable career. Julie Adams and Angie Sheard (2013) suggest tips for ensuring a healthy balance between work and 'play'. These include knowing your own limits, and 'pressing the pause button' – that means taking stock of your life, perhaps by utilising skills of reflection. It is important to listen to your body and really consider whether you should take that extra work home or not. One of the advantages of mobile technology is just that – its mobility. The number of people in the UK who work from home is rising (ONS, 2016) which makes it difficult to have a clear demarcation of where work ends and home life starts. Many people appreciate the flexibility that working from home may bring about, however, it becomes less attractive when it is in addition to the working week.

Self-care is massively important to all of us and yet becomes hugely neglected with the 24 hours-a-day lifestyle we all seem to expect and be expected to manage. In France this is recognised by many as an issue and from 2017, French companies have been required to guarantee their employees a 'right to disconnect' from technology as the country seeks to address the issues of employee burnout, brought about in part by out-of-hours email reading and responding. While it is difficult to see how this might be enforceable, it has begun a conversation about the idea of work-life balance and how employers and employees might begin to reduce the intrusion of work into people's private lives, while still maintaining and displaying a commitment to the role.

For carers, as for practitioners, the concept of resilience is in essence an idea in which they recognise what strengths they have to draw on in the face of perceived challenges, and what their values, inner strength and skills can bring to this. Being aware of *both* one's strengths and limitations is an important part of developing effective personal *and* professional resilience, and it is a capacity that can be learned as well as developed and practised. It is vital that we all work to our strengths while recognising our limitations.

There are strategies to develop and support resilience building, as well as techniques and tips that may help in this process. For example, the application of a cognitive behavioural approach (CBT) to reduce negative self-doubts that many people (carers and practitioners alike) might harbour, may be a way of helping to regulate one's emotions and enhance self-esteem and self-confidence. Mindfulness is another useful tool. Caring for oneself emotionally, physically and spiritually as well as nurturing a positive view of oneself is so important.

## Reflective **task**

Considering the points above regarding nurturing a positive view of one-self, think about the last time someone paid you a compliment. How did you respond?

Common responses may include: 'It was nothing' or 'It was just good luck' or 'I'm sure you don't mean that' or 'I don't deserve it, it was so and so's work really'. Well – STOP! Take the compliment! If your likely response appears above, think about the compliment as a physical present, a gift from that person to you – and clearly, most of us would acknowledge this gift, because to reject it would be inappropriate.

## Taking it further

1. Regarding research for practitioners, look at the following site: www.ripfa.org.uk/assets/_userfiles/files/Publications_resources/ripfa_kss_map_261016-3.pdf.

2. For an in-depth discussion regarding the Ethics of Care debate, please see Barnes, M, Brannelly, T, Ward, L and Ward, N (eds) (2015) *Ethics of Care: Critical Advances in International Perspective*. Bristol: Policy Press.

3. For further information regarding mindfulness, please see Northcutt, T B (ed) (2017) *Cultivating Mindfulness in Clinical Social Work: Narratives from Practice*. London: Springer.

# References

Adams, J and Sheard, A (2013) *Positive Social Work: The Essential Toolkit for NQSWs*. St Albans: Critical Publishing.

Aldridge, H and Hughes, C (2016) Informal carers in the UK: an analysis of the family resources survey. New Policy Institute. www.npi.org.uk/files/2114/6411/1359/Carers_and_poverty_in_the_UK_-_full_report.pdf [accessed 29 March 2018].

BASW www.basw.co.uk [accessed 10 February 2018].

Berger, J (1972) *Ways of Seeing*. Harmondsworth: Penguin.

Cairns, D, Tolson, D, Brown, J and Darbyshire, C (2013) The need for future alternatives: an investigation of the experiences and future of older parents caring for offspring with learning disabilities over a prolonged period of time. *British Journal of Learning Disabilities*, 41(1): 73–82.

Campbell, A, Taylor, B J and McGlade, A (2017) *Research Design in Social Work: Qualitative and Quantitative Methods*. London: Learning Matters.

Caplan, M A and Purser, G (2017) Qualitative inquiry using social media: a field-tested example. *Qualitative Social Work*, doi: 10.1177/1473325017725802.

Carers UK (2012) In sickness and in health: a survey of 3,400 UK carers about their health and well-being. www.carersuk.org/for-professionals/policy/policy-library?task=download&file=policy_file&id=208 [accessed 29 March 2018].

Carey, M (2013) *The Social Work Dissertation: Using Small-Scale Qualitative Methodology*. London: McGraw-Hill Education.

Dillenburger, K and McKerr, L (2011) 'How long are we able to go on?' Issues faced by older family caregivers of adults with disabilities. *British Journal of Learning Disabilities*, *39*(1): 29–38.

Emerson, E, McCulloch, A, Graham, H, Blacher, J, Llwellyn, G M and Hatton, C (2010) Socioeconomic circumstances and risk of psychiatric disorders among parents of children with early cognitive delay. *American Journal on Intellectual and Developmental Disabilities*, *115*(1): 30–42.

ESRC www.esrc.ac.uk [accessed 20 January 2018].

Fox, A, Sparrow, N and Webber, J (2010) Carers and the NHS. *British Journal of General Practice*, *60*(575): 462–3.

Gilligan, C (1982) *In a Different Voice*. Cambridge, MA: Harvard University Press.

Gilligan, R (1997) Beyond permanence? The importance of resilience in child placement practice and planning. *Adoption & Fostering*, *21*(1): 12–20.

Hardwick, L and Worsley, A (2010) *Doing Social Work Research*. London: Sage.

Howell, K (2013) *The Philosophy of Methodology*. London: Sage.

HCPC www.hcpc-uk.co.uk [accessed 20 January 2018].

Hothersall, S J (2016) Epistemology and social work: integrating theory, research and practice through philosophical pragmatism. *Social Work and Social Sciences Review*, *18*(3): 33–67.

Hughes, J and Sharrock, L (1997) *The Philosophy of Social Research* (3rd Ed). Abingdon: Routledge.

Jeffrey, J (2013) *Use of Research among Social Work Clinicians*. Master of Social Work Clinical Research Papers. Paper 201. http://sophia.stkate.edu/msw_papers/201 [accessed 20 February 2018].

Keating, N C, Fast, J E, Lero, D S, Lucas, S J and Eales, J (2014) A taxonomy of the economic costs of family care to adults. *Journal of the Economics of Ageing*, *3*: 11–20.

Kittay, E, Feder, E, and Myers, D T (eds) (1987) *Women and Moral Theory*. Lanham, MD: Rowman and Littlefield.

KSS Adults (2015) Knowledge and Skills Statement for Social Workers in Adult Services. www.gov.uk/government/uploads/system/uploads/attachment_data/file/411957/KSS.pdf [accessed 20 February 2018].

KSS Children (2014) Knowledge and skills for child and family social work. www.gov.uk/government/uploads/system/uploads/attachment_data/file/338718/140730_Knowledge_and_skills_statement_final_version_AS_RH_Checked.pdf [accessed 20 February 2018].

Li, Q and Loke, A Y (2013) The positive aspects of care-giving for cancer patients: a critical review of the literature and directions for future research. *Psycho-Oncology*, *22*(11): 2399–407.

Loi, S M, Dow, B, Moore, K, Hill, K, Russell, M, Cyarto, E, Malta, S, Ames, D and Lautenschlager, N (2016) Factors associated with depression in older carers. *International Journal of Geriatric Psychiatry*, *31*(3): 294–301.

McCann, T V, Bamberg, J and McCann, F (2015) Family carers' experience of caring for an older parent with severe and persistent mental illness. *International Journal of Mental Health Nursing*, *24*(3): 203–12.

Mayeroff, M (1971) *On Caring*. New York: Harper & Row.

Miravitlles, M, Peña-Longobardo, L M, Oliva-Moreno, J and Hidalgo-Vega, Á (2015) Care-givers' burden in patients with COPD. *International Journal of Chronic Obstructive Pulmonary Disease*, *10*: 347.

Mockford, C (2015) A review of family carers' experiences of hospital discharge for people with dementia, and the rationale for involving service users in health research. *Journal of Healthcare Leadership*, 7: 21.

NMC (2017) NMC register. www.nmc.org.uk/globalassets/sitedocuments/other-publications/nmc-register-2013-2017.pdf [accessed 9 February 2018].

ONS (2016) Homeworkers rates and levels: Jan to Mar 2015. www.ons.gov.uk/employmentandlabourmarket/peopleinwork/employmentandemployeetypes/adhocs/005578homeworkersratesandlevelsjanto mar2015 [accessed 9 February 2018].

Papastavrou, E, Kalokerinou, A, Papacostas, S S, Tsangari, H and Sourtzi, P (2007) Caring for a relative with dementia: family care-giver burden. *Journal of Advanced Nursing*, 58(5): 446–57.

Pinquart, M and Sörensen, S (2003) Associations of stressors and uplifts of caregiving with caregiver burden and depressive mood: a meta-analysis. *Journals of Gerontology Series B: Psychological Sciences and Social Sciences*, 58(2): 112–28.

Ribeiro, O and Paul, C (2008) Older male carers and the positive aspects of care. *Ageing & Society*, 28(2): 165–83.

Sage, M and Sage, T (2016) Social media and e-professionalism in child welfare: policy and practice. *Journal of Public Child Welfare*, 10(1): 79–95.

Skills for Care (2014) The state of the adult social care sector and workforce report in England, Leeds, 2015. www.skillsforcare.org.uk/stateof2014 [accessed 18 November 2017].

Stoltz, P, Udén, G and Willman, A (2004) Support for family carers who care for an elderly person at home: a systematic literature review. *Scandinavian Journal of Caring Sciences*, 18(2): 111–19.

Tronto, J C (1993) *Moral Boundaries: A Political Argument for an Ethic of Care*. London: Psychology Press.

Windle, G and Bennett, K M (2012) Caring relationships: how to promote resilience in challenging times. In *The Social Ecology of Resilience* (pp 219–31). New York: Springer.

## Chapter 7 | Young carers, older parent-carers and carers of people with dementia

This chapter will take as its focal point three distinct 'categories' of family carers; that is, carers aged 18 and under (young carers), parent-carers (over the age of 65) and carers of people with dementia. Issues faced by all three groups will be discussed. Understanding the dynamics of care and how it is organised and negotiated in families is a complex activity. Issues facing carers of all ages are different; each caring situation is unique, fluid and contextual. However, there are some similarities which may link aspects of family caring for all carers.

Highlighting some of the issues that practitioners need to be aware of in order to work effectively with young carers, carers of people with dementia and older parent-carers, this section will draw upon three case studies to highlight the points being made.

# Young carers

As a starting point to any discussion it is essential to define the terms used. What is understood by the phrase, or label, 'young carer'? How, and in what ways does being a young carer differ from just being a daughter, a son, or a brother or sister?

According to Barnardos, young carers are children who help to look after a member of the family who is sick, disabled, has mental health problems or is misusing drugs or alcohol (see www.barnardos.org.uk/what_we_do/our_work/young_carers.htm).

A more detailed and inclusive definition of what or who a young carer is has been provided by Thomas et al (2003, p 44):

*A young carer is a child or young person who is in need of specific services because their life is affected by the need to provide care for a family or household member who has an illness or disability. This may include a child or young person who provides direct personal care to another person, who takes on a supportive role for the main carer, or who undertakes domestic duties as a result of the need for care. It may also include a child or young person who is denied ordinary social or educational opportunities because of the other person's need for care. These needs may arise on a regular or occasional basis.*

As 'carers' began to become recognised as a distinct category in their own right, mainly from the 1980s onwards, so too did the notion of specific categories of family carers, most notably 'young carers' ie those carers who are children and young people under the age of 18. Recognised for the first time in the Carers (Recognition and Services) Act 1995, this extended the definition of carer to include young carer, so meaning that service providers needed to be alert to the issue of children involved in providing care.

The number of children or young people who are recognised as young carers is growing. The Office for National Statistics (ONS, 2013) figures, taken from the 2011 survey, state that there are 178,000 young carers in England and Wales, and the biggest increase was in the 5–7-year-old age group, which saw a rise of 83 per cent. The majority of young carers begins caring before the age of 12 and continues this caring throughout their childhood (Milne and Larkin, 2015).

It is important to note that these figures are likely to be influenced by a number of factors: for example, an increased awareness of the role young carers play is more likely to support their identification, and statistics are of course always open to interpretation. A BBC survey carried out in 2010, based on 4,000 secondary school pupils, estimated that the number of young carers was likely to be close to 400,000 (see www.bbc.co.uk/pressoffice/pressreleases/stories/2010/11_november/16/carers. shtml).

It is always problematic drawing generalisations from a relatively small sample based in one geographical area, and there are, of course, likely to be variations in understanding meaning attached to different questions asked in a survey. However, be that as it may, it is realistic to assume that given the current economic crisis and cuts to services, the number of family carers per se is increasing.

As noted previously in Chapter 1, caring is a hidden activity; an activity that generally takes place in private, in the confines of one's home. There may be a thin line between what is considered to be participating in 'normal' family life and the activities undertaken by young carers. Clearly, children should not have to take on caring roles merely because of a lack of alternative provision. However, there is a narrow division between what is a caring role and what are day-to-day activities of living. When does a 'young carer' become a 'young carer' and not just a child performing normal family roles? We know that some of the tasks that family carers perform include shopping, cleaning, and making meals, and clearly, in many families, it is expected that children would play their part in these tasks.

## Practical **task**

Make a list of jobs or chores that you were expected to do as a child, at a particular age – you decide when – and the frequency with which you were expected to do them.

Ask a friend or colleague to do the same. Compare the lists and consider how your experiences as a child influence what you believe is, or should be, an expected norm for participating in family life.

What seems to be a defining factor is when that 'helping' goes beyond that normally expected from children and young people of a similar age, and when the people whom they help or assist would struggle without this support. Reasons why a child or young person takes on caring responsibilities in the first place are diverse and depend, to a certain extent, on the unique structure of their family. It may be because of the need of a family member for care and support that others in the family either cannot, refuse to, or struggle to meet without additional help. It may be that there is a lack of support by the State or the wider community and that there is no one to fill the gap – apart from the young person. Definitions are problematic, as we have seen elsewhere in this book. Individual situations differ and household compositions change. There may be additional complexities when looking at the role young carers play in the lives of their family, particularly when these are not directly linked to the care of an adult in need of care and support – for example, taking care of siblings. The factors suggested above are also subject to the general conditions of society and the economy.

For many young carers, there is a subtlety and an insidiousness about the way in which care may creep up on one; for some, it may be a significant event – their parent may have a CVA and an impairment follows swiftly; whereas for others it may be the gradual decline in the mobility and cognitive ability of a grandparent. Such definitions are, of course, relative and linked to availability of other help and support. The child with a grandparent who lives in the same house may find their parents take on any necessary caring role and their own lives are relatively unaffected by the situation; for example, they may make them a drink and a snack occasionally and sit with them to read the news. Do you think this defines them as a young carer?

On the other hand they may be in a situation with just one parent living in the family home who works full time and has several other younger children to care for. This means that already there is a sense of responsibility on this young person to undertake activities perhaps to the extent to which their peers do not – laundry, shopping and cooking – as well as getting up early to make their grandparent's breakfast and help them to get dressed before they themselves go to school. It can be tricky, as it appears that many children and young people may be on the cusp of becoming young carers for family members. However, what may tip the balance is the existence or non-existence of carer-related support services that are accessible, affordable and appropriate.

Young carers are supported by legislation, namely the Children and Families Act (2014) and the Care Act (2014), with local authorities required to take reasonable steps to identify those young carers in their areas. According to Leu and Becker (2017), many of these children will be providing regular and significant amounts of care, either episodically or spread over many years, and yet they frequently remain 'hidden' from health, social care and other welfare professionals and services. All assessments of adults with care and support needs must establish if there are children involved in providing care.

Issues of the existence of and support for young carers raise a number of complex questions, particularly for practitioners.

> » Does focusing attention on, acknowledging and supporting the role young carers play in their families mean ignoring the illness or disability of the family member for whom they provide support?

> » Does funding and supporting young carers actually take away potential funding for appropriate support for the family members for whom they care?

> » If children and young people are caring for parents, is this due to a lack of alternative provision, and might it be seen as undermining the fundamental rights of parents?

Care and support needs arise from a range of different circumstances, and we know that in reality these needs are most likely to be met within the family unit. Families come in many different forms and therefore family carers will be drawn from across the age range.

What makes an exploration of issues to do with young carers so significant is that they have dual needs, both as a carer and as a young person, and the impact that caring as a child or young person may have on the trajectory of their adult life needs to be recognised. For example, as a result of their caring responsibilities young carers may miss out on opportunities other children their age have to play and learn. They may have irregular school attendance or are not punctual. When they do attend school there may be other issues such as tiredness, leading to a lack of concentration, and issues of difficulty in keeping up with school work. Research has shown how some young carers do not reveal that they are carers, and may make excuses for late or incomplete homework (Rose and Cohen, 2010). These issues have a negative impact on the academic achievement of young carers that consequently puts them at a significant disadvantage when competing in the job market.

For some young carers, school may be seen as an opportunity for a break; they have a legitimate reason to be out of the house and time to 'be' a young person. The high demands and constraints associated with many caring situations, coupled with the low level of support received by many young carers, means time at school could be seen as a welcome relief from their caring role. The lack of autonomy and freedom within a school environment, which many pupils rail against, may for many young carers be insignificant when compared to that at home, where spontaneity may be curtailed.

For some young carers, seeing their relative's vulnerability or distress, living and sharing that environment on a daily basis, may be a very stressful and pressurised situation. Being powerless to change a situation can be incredibly stressful, and to have a break from this even for just a few hours a day at school may be the only factor that enables continuation of their role.

Young carers may turn down opportunities to participate in after-school activities and trips due to pressures at home and financial constraints (as we know, caring more often than not is equated with poverty and reliance on welfare benefits). For Thomas et al (2003) young carers are doubly disadvantaged in terms of their opportunities for a social life, as they are less likely to go out with their friends because of their caring responsibilities; and because of their family's low income, they have limited opportunities for socialising and travel. Decisions about post-school options, nights out and holidays may also be curtailed as the young person might be the only one offering and/or supplying emotional support to the adult, as well as overseeing the family budget – difficult to quantify, particularly during an assessment of needs, but may be there all the same. Missing time at school is seen by many commentators as being one of the negative outcomes associated with being a young carer. However, it may be that one experience replaces another and that expertise and experience gained through caring may be seen in some way to replace, or at least support, expertise and experience gained (or lost) in education.

The limitations are not solely to do with the school or social life of a young carer, as it could be seen that other opportunities are also being curtailed – for example, the option of leaving home to attend higher or further education is constrained. For young carers who do go on to higher education, the location of the institution may be a more influential factor than the programme of study, with young carers choosing to remain living at home in order to be able to provide care for their relative. This may lead to fewer career prospects, and has implications across the life-course for career satisfaction as well as associated acquisition of savings and pension provision. Ambition to undertake further study is also affected by caring responsibilities, and it was noted by Carers Trust that 14 per cent of young carers who were at school said that they would not be able to consider going on to study at college or university because of the responsibilities of their caring role. Additionally, 24 per cent of young adult carers in school said that they did not feel they would be able to afford to go to college or university (Carers Trust https://carers.org/about-us/about-young-carers).

Being a teenager can be difficult, with many physical and emotional changes taking place, decisions needing to be made and the additional pressures of studying and possibly working. For young carers their caring responsibilities may bring an added dimension to the anxieties teenagers without caring responsibilities face – namely, worry and stress about the person for whom they care, and in the case of caring for a parent, such worries may extend to concerns about themselves – what might happen to them if their parent went into hospital or died, for example. For some teenagers there may be additional concerns regarding the illness or diagnosis of the person for whom they care, and genetic or hereditary links (Mand et al, 2015). They may be concerned about what this might mean for their own health in the future and that of any children they might have.

How are young carers identified? The terminology is problematic as it implies a family member may be in a position of dependency. As noted above, many young carers do not identify themselves as such (Smyth et al, 2011). Young carers may not know a different life without caring responsibilities or they may accept their circumstances as normal. Others may wish to keep their caring role a secret (Thomas et al, 2003). Lack of self-identity of carers is a common theme in the literature and young carers, like many other carers, remain hidden from services. As we have seen throughout this book, no element of care takes place in a vacuum. Young carers may be sons or daughters, siblings, grandchildren, nieces or nephews. As they provide care, so too should they have an adult(s) overseeing their upbringing and welfare. Their parents' capacity to keep them safe, emotionally supported, disciplined and nurtured will be influenced by a number of factors, some related to disability or impairment and associated care needs, and others not. Identification of young carers is generally made by practitioners working with the person in the family with care needs; however, schools and youth groups, as well as organisations such as scout groups also have a role to play.

Early identification of young carers is key, as is young carers themselves recognising the role they are in. Research carried out by Carers UK (2016) found that half of carers (52 per cent) in their study stated that their health was affected and half (50 per cent) said there was a negative impact on their finances because of the time it took *them* to self-identify as a carer. Clearly, there is a role for practitioners here; it is important for assessors to identify and highlight the strengths of a family, as well as identifying any challenges faced by its members, and look to ways of supporting these needs as a unit, without placing pressure on individuals within that family. Caring is a relational activity and support needs to be based on a recognition of the reciprocal nature that occurs within caring relationships.

For practitioners carrying out carers' needs assessments, it is necessary also to consider whether any of the caring tasks the child is undertaking are inappropriate and/or excessive and to document this as clearly and in as much detail as possible. It is important to remember that assessments need to be updated regularly, and assumptions made by professionals about the depth and breadth of family caring, as well as willingness and availability of family carers, may need to be challenged. Situations change and conditions – for example, mental health issues – fluctuate, just as do other conditions that mean care is needed; for example, difficulties due to motor neurone disease may worsen.

For young carers an imperceptive decline in the health or ability of their parent/family member may initially be so subtle as to go unnoticed. It becomes a new 'norm' and as such, practitioners and services are not always made aware.

## Case example

Eloise (12) lives with her Dad, Kevin, who has chronic obstructive pulmonary disease (COPD) – a progressive disease that causes increasing breathlessness, making it very difficult for Kevin to do typical day-to-day activities. He was retired early on health grounds from his job as a carpet fitter. Eloise's Mum died when she was a baby. The nearest family member is Kevin's brother Paul and his family who live in New York. As Kevin's condition has deteriorated, Eloise has done more and more for her Dad, initially just tidying up and preparing tea. However, over the past six months Eloise has had to help her Dad with some aspects of his physical care, including dressing and washing parts of his body he can't reach, as well as managing his nebuliser and oxygen supplies when he needs them.

» Make a note of what you consider the key points when carrying out an assessment for Eloise.

» What do you think may be the consequences (both negative and positive) of Eloise's role as a young carer?

For assessors, considering the family's personal histories and looking at a wide range of other factors helps to explore with young carers and their parents what their role might entail. It needs to be remembered and acknowledged that many young carers are in very different situations, and for professionals working with young carers, no two situations are the same – this sounds overly basic, but is something that needs to be restated. The interactions and dependencies that exist in families vary, and although basic human needs, for food, shelter and warmth for example, are universal, how these are approached and negotiated within families differs. Families are not all alike. Just as carers are not a homogenous group, so too young carers have many differing aspects to their lives. For example, the age of a young carer needs to be taken into account; there is a vast differential between the needs of a 6-year-old and the needs of a 15-year-old. The activities or roles they undertake may differ; they may be providing financial, physical and/or emotional support and care to a greater or lesser extent. The family member they provide care for may be a sibling, grandparent or parent, and that person's needs may differ and may come about because of a range of impairments, chronic illnesses, drug or alcohol addiction, mental health, learning or physical disability, or an emotional or behavioural issue, to name just a few examples. Other factors that need to be recognised by an assessor and professionals are that work with a family where there may be a young carer needs to have an awareness of issues, including the impact of wider society – for example, housing, employment, income, the community where the family lives and their access to wider networks of support. In practice, the knowledge a professional has of community resources and of sources of information and advice may be an important factor in arranging support to prevent a young carer from taking on the responsibility for offering a level of care that is inappropriate and/or excessive.

**Be clear**

Chris Dyke, in his excellent book *Writing Analytical Assessments in Social Work* (2016), reminds us of the need to be clear when gathering information, and the need to avoid ambiguity. Taking the example above, for instance; if you are to record that 'Eloise provides some personal care for Kevin' then think about what this might mean to other people. You are clear, but others reading that statement are unlikely to have the same understanding of 'personal care' as you do. It is far better to say what you have found out, as well as who has told you that, for example:

Eloise said she empties and cleans the commode every morning. She helps Kevin to have a wash in the evening; he is unable to reach his back and his feet, so she washes and dries them. She fetches his toothbrush, paste and a bowl twice a day and then empties them. When Kevin is struggling with his breathing, Eloise said she connects the nebuliser and stays with him, trying to help him keep calm and relaxed to help him breathe.

Are you able to see the difference?

Recording information like this takes more time initially, however it will pay off in the long run. It also helps you to demonstrate the need for services for the family and to be specific in what might best support them. It also bears witness to your asking the right sort of questions and to building a relationship with the family. As a busy practitioner, you do/will not have time to remember lots of details in your head, and if you look at an assessment you carried out 12 months earlier, are unlikely to remember the details of what you meant by 'personal care'. Being clear, recording who said what and sticking to the facts are key to being able to write high quality and useful assessments and reports.

Practitioners are criticised for using long words and trying to sound professional and academic. Remember the acronym 'KISS' – keep it simple, stupid. Adopting this to include the idea that reports and accounts within health and social care practice work best if they are kept simple rather than made complicated; simplicity should be a key goal in report writing, and unnecessary complexity should be avoided. Likewise, if you cannot understand a situation, you are unlikely to be able to explain it to others, or record it usefully, and as Dyke (2016: 71) says: 'the vocabulary doesn't make you more skillful, your skills do'.

Practitioners need to explore how they may support the adult with care needs, in order to absolve a young person from the need to provide inappropriate care. For any young person, providing intimate personal care, such as bathing and toileting, or a caring role that incorporates administering medication and physical tending, is likely to have a major impact on their own emotional and/or physical well-being, and is one that is seen as inappropriate. Similarly, the effects of long-term caring involving broken nights' sleep and potential absences from school are likely to have a long-term impact on a young person's social and personal development as well as their future prospects.

Providing care is associated with the well-being of the person with care and support needs, but also with the well-being of carers, and the physical and emotional impact of care-providing at a young age is not to be underestimated. Providing physical care – for example, lifting or moving if the person in receipt of care has mobility difficulties, may have an effect that goes beyond childhood, in terms of their own back problems. Moving equipment such as a commode or chair, or carrying heavy loads of washing may all contribute to a feeling of exhaustion, resentment and frustration. Of course, well-being is not purely measured in physical terms, and research has shown that there are positive aspects to being a young carer. Seeing caring responsibilities as contributing to part of family life and a feeling of closeness, of pulling together and of being needed, as well as being prepared for life outside the family home, are some of the examples of positive aspects of caring identified in the literature (Thomas et al, 2003). Similarly, life satisfaction, the positive effects of caring and the benefits brought about by it have also been noted (Pakenham et al, 2007).

Although the main objective of identifying and supporting young carers is to implement ways of ensuring that they are not doing too much, over and above what might be expected from a child of their age, it may be problematic when it comes to providing support. For some young carers, even if the physical and practical roles of caring for their family member are provided by an external agency, the emotional impact of caring is not abated. As suggested above, practical support may be easier to identify and easier to come by; however, emotional support for the cared-for person is not something that can be provided 'on tap' and young carers may feel that they are the only people in a position to provide this.

## Practical **task**

Make a list of five things that you feel may impact the well-being of Eloise and then of Kevin.

Now list potential ways of overcoming these – if you had a magic wand how might you approach these?

## Students as carers

This is a book aimed at a readership of health and social care students as well as at practitioners and carers, and it is worth noting that young carers as students may well make up the readership. It is a mark of the increased recognition of carers, particularly that of young carers and the nature of care in society, that a campaign initiated by a student carer has recently been adopted by the Universities and Colleges Admissions Services (UCAS) (see https://carers.org/news-item/ucas-form-identify-student-carers).

As noted elsewhere in this book, identification is key, and this is particularly pertinent in terms of providing support for young carers who are at university. First of all, universities need to know of their existence. In the UK from 2018 there will be a specific option on the university application form for carers to acknowledge themselves as such. This will help universities to identify whether applicants would be studying as well as providing unpaid care for someone with an illness, disability, mental health problem or an addiction. Second, universities need to be able to act on this information and ensure awareness, information and understanding is available to students who have additional responsibilities. Some universities have bursaries for young carers, some have support groups; however, an overall awareness is key to good practice. Some 49 per cent of young people now attend university (www.theguardian.com/education/2017/sep/28/almost-half-of-all-young-people-in-england-go-on-to-higher-education), and many of these will be young carers.

Carers Trust (https://carers.org/about-us/about-young-carers) has identified that half of young adult carers in college or university are struggling because of their caring role. Students may be tired, lack concentration, or struggle to attend lectures that may be timed later or earlier in the day than they were previously used to with school hours. Students who are young carers may already have many relevant life skills, including time management, multi-tasking and working as a team, as well as budgeting and they will have a lot to offer universities as well as future employers. For colleges and universities, the level of support offered to young carers may be key to retaining them throughout their programme of study. Flexibility and understanding, as well as peer support, are important factors to help young carers achieve their potential as students. Carers Trust noted that young adult carers are four times more likely to have dropped out of college or university than students without caring roles. Given the cost of tuition fees in English universities, leaving without a degree has financial implications on future debt and lack of earnings and the act of dropping out may have repercussions on the self-esteem and confidence of the young person, as well as changing the nature of their relationship with the person for whom they care.

*If you are reading this book as a student, think for a moment about who most people talk to if they are having a stressful time. Friendships made at university can be life-long, and friends play a key role in supporting each other through difficult times. Start a conversation. Today.

# Older parent-carers of adults with learning difficulties

This section will focus on a different demographic of family carers – that of older parent-carers. As babies and children with complex disabilities are living longer, being a parent of someone with a learning difficulty may be a lifelong commitment. It is possible to see that becoming a parent of a son or daughter with a learning difficulty alters people's lives in many different ways. It has major significance for personal biographies; experiences and perceptions are shaped by the cultural and social context in which these parents live their lives. Many parents may feel they face a lifetime of caring responsibilities (Kim et al, 2003) and the presence of a child with a disability within a family can be a turning point in the parents' biography (Chamberlayne and King, 1997). This group of carers is particularly interesting, as the longevity of the caring experience may, as suggested, last for decades. Other carers may move in and out of caring; however, parents of children (and then adults), with learning difficulties, are generally in it for the 'long(est) haul'.

For many parent-carers, misunderstandings about the ability of their son or daughter and about the term 'independent living' may have been formed decades ago (Foundation for People with Learning Disabilities, 2002). As with many aspects of development for adults with learning disabilities, problems arise when parents reflect on the information they were given when their son or daughter's diagnosis of learning difficulty was first made (Lovell and Mason, 2012).

Think about this for a moment: perhaps you can recall a comment made to you by a family member, friend, or colleague that you have 'held' on to, only to mention it later and be greeted by bemusement.

For many carers those in 'authority' with power and access to services have a profound effect on their lives. Often a throwaway comment can be the cause of much discussion, debate and potential anxiety for carers, and for some carers if they were told something in their formative caring years about the ability or life expectation/ chances or opportunities for their loved one, they may hold on to that fact throughout their lifetime.

People are proud and want to be seen to be coping. Often caring will earn the admiration of others, including friends and neighbours, who may occasionally wonder how the carer copes; this 'raising up' on a pedestal of carers in some circumstances makes it even more difficult for carers to admit that they can't manage any longer.

With parents such as those mentioned in the 'I'm not a nurse, but' campaign in Chapter 4, the specifics of the impairment of their son or daughter has not surprisingly shaped the role and type of care provided. There is no one typical situation of providing care, just as there is no one particular type of disability. Generalisations can be drawn within diagnoses such as cerebral palsy, epilepsy, Down's syndrome, autism, etc. However, within these diagnoses there is such a broad spectrum of ability and need that makes generalisations of their situations difficult.

Focusing on older parent-carers of adults with learning difficulties enables an exploration of key areas of support and guidance that will be pertinent for all (older) carers. Although the peak age for caring is 50–64 there are approximately 1.3 million people over the age of 65 who provide care in England and Wales (Carers UK, 2015). These carers will include adult children providing care for their parents, and spouses caring for each other. One small but growing minority among those carers aged 65+ are carers of adults with disabilities. Although the number of carers is increasing, many people move in and out of caring, and there is a fluidity with those people caring now being less likely to do so in five years. For parent-carers of adults with learning difficulties, providing practical, physical and emotional care may have been the situation for decades, along with the associated emotional, physical and financial implications (Walker and Ward, 2013; Carers UK 2015).

As noted in Chapter 1 the survival into adulthood of people with some very complex physical and cognitive difficulties means that many parents may experience a lifetime of caring. People with learning difficulties in particular are living longer and, as research indicates, the majority of people with learning disabilities live with their families; this means that many of these family carers will be elderly people.

Some of the challenges faced by this group of older parent-carers will be discussed below.

Adults with learning difficulties continue to live longer in an increasingly ageing population and it is notable that for the first time, people with learning difficulties are surviving into old age in significant numbers. Emerson and Hatton (2008) forecast that growth in numbers of adults of 60 years and over with learning difficulties could increase as much as 50 per cent by 2021; and there continues to be huge growth in this demographic of older parent-carers. As stated above, most adults with learning difficulties live with their families, and family carers (usually parent(s)) are themselves ageing and many are unknown to services. Literature indicates that many carers continue to feel invisible and ignored, without due recognition for the important role they perform both within their family and within society at large.

What are the experiences of older parent-carers, and how might these be used to inform health and social care practitioners' practice with carers? Many older parent-carers have decades of experience of caring for their son or daughter, generally from birth to old age. The lives of all parties become entwined and interdependent with reciprocity of care, both emotional and practical, as well as a joint financial base becoming the norm.

## Case example

Molly and Harry have been married for 55 years; they are both in their 80s, and have two children, Jack and Karen. Harry retired from his job when he was 58 due to ill health; he has mobility problems and experiences almost constant pain in his back. Molly gave up work when she had Jack. She is in excellent physical health, although admits to becoming more forgetful, and is currently undergoing assessment at a memory clinic.

Their older child, Jack, is 53 and works for HMRC (Her Majesty's Revenue and Customs). He lives with his wife, Jennie, a nurse, and their three teenage sons in a city 50 miles away from his parents.

Karen (Molly and Harry's daughter) is 46 and lives at home with her parents. She has Down's syndrome and epilepsy. Until recently Karen attended a local day centre for adults with disabilities. This recently closed and Karen is now in receipt of a personal budget that enables her to go swimming and to attend a city farm with a support worker three times a week.

» Make a note of the name(s) of the family carer(s) in the above account.

» What do you consider to be the main areas of responsibility for them?

» How long do you think the care in this situation might have been provided for?

» What was it about the information that made you think that?

One of the most significant factors in older carer families is the mutually dependent relationship that exists between the adult with a learning difficulty and their older parent-carer. If you noted that Harry or Molly were carers in the above case study, you would not be wrong. As parents they will undoubtedly have gained years of experience of caring for and supporting Karen, through health and social care assessments and with certain aspects of daily life. However, over decades there may be evidence to support the fact that the family has become a trio, with Karen also carrying out a caring role, supporting her parents both physically and emotionally. Consider for a moment: if you were carrying out an assessment as a health and social care practitioner, would you consider offering Karen an assessment in her own right as a carer?

It may be the case for older parent-carers and their sons or daughters that both caregiving and care-receiving are their 'norm'. A major challenge for older parent-carers is that of the future – planning ahead is key for older families where there is a son or daughter who has a learning difficulty. Many parents of people with learning difficulties say that they have no definite plans if and when a time comes when they are unable to continue caring for their offspring. Many carers of people with a learning difficulty say that they are anxious about the future (Gant, 2010; Cairns et al, 2013) and require more support, advice and information from professionals, who in turn need to show greater awareness of people's concerns (Cairns et al, 2013; Carers UK, 2015).

It would seem obvious that being proactive is better than being reactive. For a busy practitioner, forward planning with an older carer is better than last-minute crisis involvement following their death or emergency hospitalisation resulting in their son or daughter having to be placed as an emergency, losing their routine, their home and the person with whom they have lived with all their life in one fell swoop. In the long term, prevention services will be less costly: financially and emotionally.

It can be a challenge for older parents of adults with learning difficulties to recognise that they need to face up to the future. Years of experience in dealing with professionals may have left parents with a less than optimistic view about what organisations are actually able to do to support them, and impressions formed about their own son or daughter's ability – based on professional opinion perhaps expressed decades ago – have a resonance in the present. Families need to be seen as co-experts, with their views respected and listened to. This presents a challenge for practitioners in ensuring that parents' views do not obscure the views and wishes of the person with a learning difficulty. Skill and experience are needed to ensure that both voices are heard and recorded. Understanding contemporary issues is vital for practice and further exploration is needed regarding how professionals integrate various types of knowledge in order to strengthen practice.

Another challenge that may be experienced by older parent-carers is a financial one. We know that carers are more likely to experience poverty and hardship than those without caring responsibilities. Likewise, the implications of providing care for decades will have an impact on savings and pension contributions. In addition to the physical, emotional and practical elements of reciprocal care, there may be an economic element. The various benefits people receive – for example, personal independence payments paid to the adult with a learning difficulty – might have become an intrinsic part of the general household income and it can be a challenge trying to separate this out.

## Case example continued

It is now two years later. Harry's mobility has worsened to such an extent that he has moved to a care home. Molly is 'just about managing' to stay in the family home and she and Karen have been looking after each other. Jack has reduced his hours at work and has been helping to support his parents and sister, particularly with attending health appointments and managing the paperwork associated with Karen's personal budget.

Karen is now 48 and has recently stated that she wants to leave home and go to live with her boyfriend, Andrew, whom she met at the farm. She says she loves him and wants to have a baby.

» Considering the above, what do you think are the issues and implications of Karen's statement?

» Do you think there is a role for professionals here?

» If so, why, and who might be involved?

» If not, why do you think that might be, and what are you basing that decision on?

» If you were to identify who is now a carer, has your view changed?

A challenge for practitioners, when working with any family within which there is a caring scenario, is to unpick the subtleties and nuances of who is providing care. We have seen that caring is relational and in many cases reciprocal. However, financial benefits and policies allied to the welfare system tend to take a lateral approach, requiring the construction of one person as 'the carer' and one person as 'the cared-for'. As well as the wider implications of this approach, there are specific implications for all concerned, particularly if an adult with a learning difficulty expresses a desire to move on, as parent-carers may be so dependent on the 'household' income that in some instances, without it they may be unable to survive financially. Changes that affect one family member have an impact on others. The scenario of parent-care-giver and adult-care-recipient is not mutually exclusive. As Fine and Glendinning (2005) have suggested, care is not a situation where an active care-giver performs an activity on a passive and dependent recipient; as such, it is important to recognise that the needs of all parties in the relationship must be taken into account when planning for the future. The issue of reciprocity within the nexus of the family structure has the potential to be easily overlooked, particularly given the interlocking nature of other issues. It should be noted that the clear presence of reciprocity of care within the broader family relationship may often be one of the most sizeable barriers to planning for the future, as the components inherent within it are not reducible to their elemental parts; the whole is clearly greater than the sum of its parts (Bowey and McGlaughlin, 2006). The impact of spending cuts has an impact on the provision of care across the sector, and for adults with disabilities who may wish to move out of their parents' homes, options may also be limited because of this.

# Caring for adults with dementia

As previously noted, the rise in demand for informal family care has never been greater and is expected to continue. Increases in longevity, coupled with technological advances, mean that the population of 'old' 'old' will continue to rise, with associated health and emotional issues that impact not only on individuals but also on those around them.

Dementia is a general term for a decline in mental ability severe enough to interfere with daily life. The two major types of dementia are (a) Alzheimer's, which is a type of dementia that causes problems with memory, thinking and behaviour. Symptoms usually develop slowly and get worse over time, becoming severe enough to interfere with daily tasks; and (b) vascular dementia, which occurs following strokes that block major brain blood vessels.

Caring for adults with dementia and associated conditions is expected to place unsustainable demands on health and social care services, according to a report published by the World Health Organization (WHO, 2017). Launching the first global monitoring system for dementia, the WHO notes that the costs globally of funding services to care for people with dementia will cost US$2 trillion in little over a decade. The WHO estimates that the number of people with dementia will reach 152 million by 2050 (current estimates globally are 50 million, so a three-fold increase as the 'baby boomers' of the 1950s and 1960s approach their centenary). The WHO notes that dementia is also overwhelming for the families and carers of those affected by it. Behavioural problems that may be exhibited by someone with dementia may be difficult for carers to manage. Features of dementia include restlessness, an inability to converse, agitation, aggression and not recognising the carer. Changes in personality may be particularly difficult to manage, especially for spousal carers, many of whom may have been together for decades. Stress is caused to families by pressures including physical, emotional and economic pressures and support is required from the health, social, financial and legal systems. With such an ageing population and as yet no cure or prevention, dementia is likely to become the twenty-first century's biggest killer.

## Case example

Jane, a 79-year-old retired secretary, is a widow with two children, Gary (49) and Nicole (51). Jane lives alone in a town in the north east of England and was diagnosed with Alzheimer's disease two years ago. The disease progressed slowly and Jane has been able to manage, with support from Nicole, together with her own sisters aged 77 and 75. Gary lives in New Zealand and keeps in regular contact by telephone and post as well as using Skype, when he knows his sister will be at the family home.

Two months ago Nicole received a telephone call at 3am from the police advising that Jane had been taken to the police station after a member of the public had found her in a distressed state, wearing her only her pyjamas and slippers. Jane had told the police that she was 'going to the shop to buy bread for Mum'. Luckily she had her purse with her which contained Nicole's details.

Following this episode it was agreed that Nicole would move into her Mum's house from Monday to Friday. Paid carers were appointed to cover the weekends. This situation continued for several weeks until one of the weekend carers failed to turn up. Nicole phoned Gary in New Zealand sobbing and saying that she 'couldn't do this any longer'. She admitted to Gary that she had screamed at Jane in anger after Jane had spilt a cup of coffee and had then attempted to clean the spill using Nicole's freshly ironed dress.

You are newly appointed to the team, and have been allocated Jane and Nicole to work with. Gary telephones you in your office at 9am on Monday; he is worried and upset about the emotional health of his sister and concerned for his Mum's safety.

» Considering the above scenario, what do you think are the main issues?

» Do you think there needs to be a safeguarding concern raised?

» If so why, and who might be involved?

> » If not, why do you think that might be and what are you basing that decision on?
>
> » How would you prioritise what actions you might take?

Caring for someone with progressive dementia is not easy. Dementia can be a complex and very unpredictable condition. As the disease progresses, the amount of care that needs to be provided in order to enable the person with dementia to manage everyday life is likely to increase (Carers Trust https://carers.org/supporting-carers-people-dementia). This is a complex area. Research literature (Livingston et al, 2010) indicates that adults with dementia are at risk of abuse from (among others) their family carers. Carers' abusive behaviour (Cooper et al, 2010) is not always easy to identify and, of course, it is inexcusable. Stress, exhaustion, a lack of choice in terms of one's hoped-for life trajectory, infused with moral and familial imperatives may contribute to and precipitate abusive behaviour. It would be naive for practitioners not to envisage this. Issues of safeguarding have been discussed elsewhere in this text; however, practitioners need to be cognisant of the possibility of abuse, harm or neglect on both sides of the caring/cared-for equation.

This section has looked at aspects of three different areas of family care-giving: young carers, older parent-carers and carers of people with dementia, and has noted issues of education for young carers, including those young carers who may be university students. Regarding older parent-carers of adults with disabilities, this section has focused on planning for the future for older parent-carers. Through the use of case studies this chapter has attempted to highlight some areas for practitioners to be aware of. With regard to carers of people with dementia, this section looked at some of the key facts about the predicted rise in numbers of people who will be diagnosed with dementia and some of the issues of abuse, harm and neglect.

Ideas for working with family carers of all ages are included in Box 1.

## Box 1

Ways of working with family carers:

» Share information – be aware of current options.

» Listen, assess and respond.

» Work in partnership.

» Be proactive – don't expect carers to come to you.

» Support and prepare before meetings or presentations – do your homework.

» Acknowledge and value the work that carers do.

» Consider ways of offering education and training (for example pain management, dealing with dementia, etc).

» Start the conversation – no one expects you to have all the answers.

This chapter has introduced you to the concept of 'care' as it relates specifically to three groups of carers. While recognising that every caring situation is unique, there are some similarities between carers; however, there are also specific characteristics that differentiate each 'group'. Using case study examples to highlight key points, this chapter also considers issues relating to students as carers and ways of supporting them to achieve their potential. This chapter emphasises the importance of clear and detailed recording by practitioners and of agencies working together in order to support both the carer and the person in receipt of care, fairly and successfully.

## Taking it further

For more information regarding the services for young carers, look at the following sites.

www.actionforchildren.org.uk/what-we-do/children-young-people/supporting-young-carers/.

www.childline.org.uk/info-advice/home-families/family-relationships/young-carers/.

For older people you may also be interested in www.ageuk.org.uk/globalassets/age-uk/documents/information-guides/ageukig13_advice_for_carers_inf.pdf.

For people with dementia and their carers

www.scie.org.uk/dementia/resources/files/working-in-partnership-with-carers.pdf.

# References

Bowey, L and McGlaughlin, A (2006) Older carers of adults with a learning disability confront the future: issues and preferences in planning. *British Journal of Social Work, 37*(1): 39–54.

Cairns, D, Tolson, D, Brown, J and Darbyshire, C (2013) The need for future alternatives: an investigation of the experiences and future of older parents caring for offspring with learning disabilities over a prolonged period of time. *British Journal of Learning Disabilities, 41*(1): 73–82.

Carers Trust (a) About young carers. https://carers.org/about-us/about-young-carers [accessed 10 February 2018].

Carers Trust (b) Supporting carers of people with dementia. https://carers.org/supporting-carers-people-dementia [accessed 10 February 2018].

Carers UK (2015) *Valuing Carers 2015 – the Rising Value of Carers' Support.* University of Sheffield, University of Leeds and CIRCLE, published by Carers UK.

Carers UK (2016) Missing out: the identification challenge. www.carersuk.org/for-professionals/policy/policy-library/missing-out-the-identification-challenge [accessed 29 March 2018].

Chamberlayne, P and King, A (1997) The biographical challenge of caring. *Sociology of Health & Illness, 19*(5): 601–21.

Cooper, C, Blanchard, M, Selwood, A, Walker, Z and Livingston, G (2010) Family carers' distress and abusive behaviour: longitudinal study. *British Journal of Psychiatry, 196*(6): 480–5.

Dyke, C (2016) *Writing Analytical Assessments in Social Work.* St Albans: Critical Publishing.

Emerson, E and Hatton, C (2008) CEDR research report 2008 (1): People with learning disabilities in England.

Fine, M and Glendinning, C (2005) Dependence, independence or interdependence? Revisiting the concepts of 'care' and 'dependency'. *Ageing & Society, 25*(4): 601–21.

Foundation for People with Learning Disabilities (2002) Preparing for the future: people with learning disabilities and their ageing family carers, *3*(13).

Gant, V (2010) Older carers and adults with learning disabilities: stress and reciprocal care. *Mental Health and Learning Disabilities Research and Practice, 7*(2): 159–72.

Kim, H W, Greenberg, J S, Seltzer, M M and Krauss, M W (2003) The role of coping in maintaining the psychological well-being of mothers of adults with intellectual disability and mental illness. *Journal of Intellectual Disability Research, 47*(4–5): 313–27.

Leu, A and Becker, S (2017) A cross-national and comparative classification of in-country awareness and policy responses to 'young carers'. *Journal of Youth Studies, 20*(6): 750–62.

Livingston, G, Leavey, G, Manela, M, Livingston, D, Rait, G, Sampson, E, Bavishi, S, Shahriyamolki, K and Cooper, C (2010) Making decisions for people with dementia who lack capacity: qualitative study of family carers in UK. *British Medical Journal, 341*: 4184.

Livingston, G, Barber, J, Rapaport, P, Knapp, M, Griffin, M, King, D, Livingston, D, Mummery, C, Walker, Z, Hoe, J and Sampson, E L (2013) Clinical effectiveness of a manual based coping strategy programme (START, STrAtegies for RelaTives) in promoting the mental health of carers of family members with dementia: pragmatic randomised controlled trial. *British Medical Journal, 347*: 6276.

Lovell, A and Mason, T (2012) Caring for a child with a learning disability born into the family unit: women's recollections over time. *Scandinavian Journal of Disability Research, 14*(1): 15–29.

Mand, C M, Gillam, L, Duncan, R E and Delatycki, M B (2015) 'I'm scared of being like mum': the experience of adolescents living in families with Huntington's disease. *Journal of Huntington's Disease, 4*(3): 209–17.

Milne, A and Larkin, M (2015) Knowledge generation about care-giving in the UK: a critical review of research paradigms. *Health & Social Care in the Community, 23*(1): 4–13.

ONS (Office for National Statistics) (2013) ONS 2011 Census analysis: unpaid care in England and Wales, 2011 and comparison with 2001. www.ons.gov.uk/ons/dcp171766_300039.pdf [accessed 3 November 2017].

Pakenham, K I, Chiu, J, Bursnall, S and Cannon, T (2007) Relations between social support, appraisal and coping and both positive and negative outcomes in young carers. *Journal of Health Psychology*, *12*(1): 89–102.

Rose, H D and Cohen, K (2010). The experiences of young carers: a meta-synthesis of qualitative findings. *Journal of Youth Studies*, 13(4): 473–87.

Smyth, C, Blaxland, M and Cass, B (2011) 'So that's how I found out I was a young carer and that I actually had been a carer most of my life'. Identifying and supporting hidden young carers. *Journal of Youth Studies*, *14*(2): 145–60.

Thomas, N, Stainton, T, Jackson, S, Cheung, W Y, Doubtfire, S and Webb, A (2003) 'Your friends don't understand': invisibility and unmet need in the lives of young carers. *Child & Family Social Work*, *8*(1): 35–46.

Walker, C and Ward, C (2013) Growing older together: ageing and people with learning disabilities and their family carers. *Tizard Learning Disability Review*, *18*(3): 112–19.

WHO (World Health Organization) (2017) *Global action plan on the public health response to dementia 2017–2025*. Geneva: World Health Organization. Licence: CC BY-NC-SA 3.0 IGO.

## Chapter 8 | Reflections and conclusion: Looking to the future

This chapter will summarise the key themes, issues and debates raised in earlier chapters to allow us to consider and discuss what the future may hold for family carers, caring and those being cared for. This chapter looks particularly at issues relating to safeguarding vulnerable adults. We are all vulnerable at some points in our lives and in need of care and support; however, a safeguarding enquiry is a specific and different process from a needs assessment, although there are similarities (Feldon, 2017). Changes brought about by the Care Act (2014) have highlighted the role of local authorities in undertaking safeguarding enquiries and these will be noted within this chapter.

Issues relating to 'post' caring, and in particular those to do with carers and loss, are discussed. For many carers existential matters abound and this chapter will offer for consideration some points of discussion in relation to carers and spirituality.

As emphasised throughout this book, care-giving and receiving is likely to touch us all personally at some point, and for those working in the health and social care professions, it is more than likely to touch us professionally on an increasingly regular basis. We might wish to remind ourselves again what Kleinman (2012, p 1550) so eloquently stated in Chapter 1:

*Care-giving is one of the foundational moral meanings and practices in human experience everywhere: it defines human value and resists crude reduction to counting and costing.*

The chapter concludes with some examples of work that is happening with carers throughout the UK and offers suggestions for practitioners in how to take forward learning from this book

# Safeguarding

Safeguarding is everyone's concern. For practitioners working in health and social care an understanding of the issue of safeguarding is a must. The duty of local authorities to undertake safeguarding enquiries has been described as a major provision of the 2014 Care Act (Feldon, 2017). There are six key principles underpinning safeguarding work.

(a) Empowerment – *Person-led decisions and informed consent.*

(b) Prevention – *Better to take action before harm occurs.*

(c) Proportionality – *Proportionate and the least intrusive response appropriate to the risk presented.*

(d) Protection – *Support and representation for those in greatest need.*

(e) Partnership – *Local solutions through services working with their communities. Communities have a part to play in preventing, detecting and reporting neglect and abuse.*

(f) Accountability – *Accountability and transparency in delivering safeguarding.*

Carers have a key role in issues of safeguarding: they may be the 'alerter' of harm or abuse. They may be the receiver of harm or abuse (intentional or unintentional) from the person whom they support or from an organisation or professional with whom they are in contact. They may be the perpetrator of harm or neglect (intentional or unintentional) of the adults they support, either on their own or with others. It is important for practitioners to be clear about the process of a safeguarding enquiry (often called a section 42 enquiry, as this duty is set out in section 42 of the Care Act) and to be aware of their responsibilities, and those of their agency or organisation.

## Safeguarding enquiries: Section 42 of the Care Act 2014

Section 42 applies where a local authority has reasonable cause to suspect that

(1) An adult in its area (whether or not ordinarily resident there)

(a) has needs for care and support (whether or not the authority is meeting any of those needs);

(b) is experiencing, or is at risk of, abuse or neglect;

(c) as a result of those needs is unable to protect himself or herself against the abuse or neglect or the risk of it;

(2) The local authority must make (or cause to be made) whatever enquiries it thinks necessary to enable it to decide whether any action should be taken in the adult's case (whether under this Part or otherwise) and, if so, what and by whom.

(3)  'Abuse' includes financial abuse; and for that purpose 'financial abuse' includes

(a)  having money or other property stolen;

(b)  being defrauded;

(c)  being put under pressure in relation to money or other property;

(d)  having money or other property misused.

(Feldon, 2017)

An initial enquiry is made following a safeguarding concern reported to the local authority. This concern may be reported by anyone, and may be anonymous. If the criteria are met and the adult consents to an enquiry taking place (or if not, there is appropriate reason for setting aside consent) then the local authority decides which organisation will lead the enquiry. The next stage of the process is for an enquiry plan to be developed which sets out who will do what, how it will be reported on, and the timescales involved. The safeguarding enquiry itself establishes the desired outcomes of the adult concerned and ensures that these are fully considered. Views of others – family and friends – are heard and involvement of others, for example, an independent advocate, and other agencies are obtained. An account of the concern is heard, whether that is to do with an individual or an agency. Additionally, the police may be involved, if appropriate. A conclusion is drawn as to whether neglect and/or abuse has taken place, and a safeguarding plan is then developed.

## Safeguarding Adults Board

Since the inception of the Care Act, local authorities are obliged to set up a Safeguarding Adults Board (SAB). The main purpose of an SAB is to assure itself that local safeguarding arrangements are in place as defined by the Care Act 2014 and statutory guidance. Some of the SAB's duties are to:

» Carry out safeguarding adult reviews

» Develop preventative strategies working collaboratively to prevent abuse and neglect where possible

» Identify the role, responsibility, authority and accountability of agencies, professional groups and individuals

» Assuring itself that safeguarding practice is monitored and reviewed.

For a complete list of SAB duties please see the Care Act (2014 §43).

## Safeguarding Adults Reviews

Section 44 of the Care Act (2014) highlights the need for a Safeguarding Adults Review (SAR) to be held when an adult in the area dies or experiences serious abuse or neglect and there is concern that partner agencies might have worked more effectively to protect the adult.

In essence the purpose of an SAR is to promote learning and improve practice, not to reinvestigate a case or to apportion blame. The objectives include establishing:

> » lessons that can be learned from how professionals and their agencies work together;
>
> » how effective the safeguarding procedures are;
>
> » how to learn and share good practice issues;
>
> » how to identify ways to improve local inter-agency practice;
>
> » how to identify ways of improving services or development needs for one or more service or agency.

Safeguarding concerns arise within and across a range of circumstances, and there is much evidence in the literature about people in receipt of care who are harmed by those caring *for* them; both family carers and those providing care in paid positions, in both domestic and residential settings (care homes and the like) (Yan, 2014; Selwood et al, 2009; Cooney et al, 2006.).

There is however *significantly less* research and evidence regarding harm and abuse occasioned upon carers by the people being *cared for*. Families may find it difficult to discuss their experiences, and feel ashamed to admit that such things actually occur. Such reasoning may arise because of the fear of blame, perhaps even prosecution or other negative consequences, such as the cared-for person moving or being (statutorily) removed from the family home. They may also find it difficult to raise concerns over the care of their family members who are in residential care for fear that, if they are wrong, they may jeopardise the place of their loved one. Because it is such a sensitive and a (largely) hidden area, it is likely to be difficult to broach with people.

By practitioners developing knowledge and skills of working with family carers, and recognising that such situations *do* exist, harm reduction strategies can be developed, and the needs of all those involved brought to the fore without the damaging effects of labelling, stigma and intense anxiety. Practitioners need to be aware that these situations are very real for some people, and respond accordingly and, importantly, proportionately (Vaddadi et al, 2002). Additionally, practitioners need to be alert to the possibility of harm and abuse happening at any time and in any family relationship, and much could be learned from the literature on child-to-adult violence (Holt, 2016) to help inform our thinking on what appears to be a common, but deeply hidden phenomenon that has the potential to affect large numbers of people (Cooper et al, 2009; Walsh and Krienert, 2007; Tyrer et al, 2006).

Working with family carers can be exciting, innovative, complex, and at times frustrating. There are many examples of excellent projects and pieces of work throughout the UK to support the work that family care-givers undertake. Examples of these include:

» Carers' cards or 'passports': these are schemes offering carers discounts and concessions at various retail and leisure venues when they show a voucher or token.

» Carer emergency cards: carers may worry about what would happen in an emergency, and some areas offer those carers registered with the carers centre a free, pocket-sized card that can be carried as a source of identification in the event of accident or illness. The registration and telephone numbers on the card are linked to a database where help can be coordinated to assist the person in receipt of care while the carer is receiving attention.

» Another innovation that may benefit carers is the charity organisation, The Lions' 'Message in a Bottle Scheme', which encourages people to keep personal and medical details in a bottle in the fridge. If a carer had an accident, or sudden illness, then the emergency services know where they can find the information that they need. They are alerted by a sticker on the front door of the property and one on the fridge.

» Carer initiatives also include a variety of activities on offer at carers centres – for example, reminiscence groups for people with dementia and their carers to attend together.

» Some centres have schemes especially for siblings and young carer activities that may run throughout the school holidays.

» Some carers centres run 'carer gardens'; this is an allotment where carers are invited to join in with planting and growing, or simply to use it as a space to sit and reflect.

» Singing groups and pampering sessions are also examples of innovations available at some carers centres.

What is needed is for practitioners to be aware of what is available. This might be as simple as putting people in touch with a local carers centre, but having some background knowledge of the services offered and even 'testimonials' from other carers who have used such services may be really helpful. It is important to recognise that services for carers are delivered elsewhere. While carers centres are an excellent resource, other organisations can and do take carer involvement seriously. One example of this is involving carers in the 'arts'. Participation in the creative arts is increasingly recognised as a source of well-being for carers and for the person for whom they care (Walsh et al, 2004; Roberts et al, 2011). There is a variety of methods that may be used, particularly by arts therapists, who involve the use of viewing and creating art, drama, music and dance/movement in a therapeutic way in order to enhance the well-being of both the carer and the person in receipt of care; and research has identified the potential for enhancing carer well-being through arts therapies (Weatherup, 2008). For practitioners considering and being open to suggesting and embracing new initiatives designed to support and enhance the caring role, thinking creatively opens up huge possibilities. There is a growing body of research evidence that indicates the benefits which use of the arts in cultural heritage centres and, in particular, museums and galleries, might bring to the health and well-being of the communities they serve (Camic and Chatterjee, 2013).

Such cultural heritage centres work with specific audiences through targeted programmes; for example, in Manchester, Manchester Museums and Galleries had an established programme of health and well-being initiatives and projects, including 'Who Cares?' This was a health and well-being project that ran for two years (2009–11) supported by health professionals, researchers, and six museums across North West England, and which included a therapeutic space providing a stimulus for curiosity, exploration, reflection and meditation. Such initiatives contribute to the well-being and resilience of individuals, including of course, carers (www2.le.ac.uk/departments/museumstudies/rcmg/publications/mind-body-spirit-report).

The idea of promoting 'social capital' as a way of working with family carers is one which may be useful for practitioners to consider. There are obvious limitations for practitioners – for example, while you may be aware of and believe in the efficacy of art therapy, there is a seriously underfunded provision; a shortage of trained specialist arts therapists and the associated costs inhibit involvement in many cases. Projects may be short term and reliant on the enthusiasm and passion of individual members of staff to drive such initiatives forward. In spite of this, it remains an area that may be useful for practitioners to be aware of in order to enhance carer well-being. More and more art galleries and museums are opening up to the possibilities there are for them to engage with the health and overall well-being of individuals; this obviously includes carers and the person for whom care is provided. Museums and galleries are public forums, generally free to enter, and can bring about benefits to health and well-being of society per se as well as addressing issues faced by many carers, specifically including social isolation (Dodd, 2002).

Practitioners working with carers need to appreciate that how society views health and well-being is changing. Well-being is not solely linked to economic prosperity (Atkinson et al, 2016), but is a complex and multifaceted phenomenon. If we take a definition of well-being as the one provided in 2011 by No Health without Mental Health we see that well-being is:

A positive state of mind and body, feeling safe and able to cope, with a sense of connection with people, communities and the wider environment.

('No Health without Mental Health', 2011)

How, then, might practitioners work to ensure that these are the goals for achieving their work with carers?

Carers are often an undervalued group and while caring for someone can be rewarding, it can also take a toll on the carer's health and well-being. Carers' needs can go unacknowledged and carers rarely demand access to psychological therapies.

The community arts therapies project developed the idea of providing arts therapies taster days for carers to test whether engaging in arts therapies could benefit well-being by being both healing and restorative. In doing so, this fits with the same key theme in the Department of Health policy:

*'Well-being: A positive state of mind and body, feeling safe and able to cope, with a sense of connection with people, communities and the wider environment.'*

(HM Government, 2011)

# Post-caring: Carers and loss

All of us experience loss during our lifetime. It is important to note that loss and grief arise not only through death and bereavement, but also from a range of other losses. Although being a carer opens up new experiences and possibilities, it is true to say that it may also bring with it loss and grief. The life you envisaged for yourself and your loved one is no more. As Hugh Marriot (2003) suggests, loss and grief are associated with the loss of both the person you knew and the relationship you once had with them and not just with death and bereavement. For many carers these losses go unrecognised, unacknowledged and unarticulated, but that does not diminish their impact. Loss may also incorporate loss of a career, of friends, of a planned and anticipated life, of the future dreamed of.

As discussed in Chapter 6 carers need to be resilient, and need a 'thick skin' to be out in public. However, for many carers that skin becomes as fragile as gossamer after decades of supporting and promoting your family member or friend's well-being and human rights, as well as your own, and it is one which may be difficult to sustain.

## Case example

Linda and Dave have been married for 23 years. They have always had what Linda describes as a 'volatile relationship' and have separated on several occasions. They have two children, Emma (aged 19 and living away from home at university) and Michael, aged 21. Michael was on his way to work when he was involved in a road traffic accident between his motorbike and a lorry. He sustained severe head injuries and after a long period in hospital and rehabilitation is now living back at home. As well as the physical effects of the accident, including seizures and partial paralysis, Michael has cognitive and intellectual impairments, memory loss and poor concentration. He needs a lot of support with most of the tasks of daily living, including personal care. He has limited speech and experiences acute anxiety when he is alone in a room. Paid carers attend twice a day to support him with washing and dressing, however, the majority of care is provided by his parents.

Linda said Dave refuses to talk about his feelings, and that one night he broke down and says he 'can't do this any more'. All he wants to do is to 'take Michael for a pint and for things to be the way they were'. Linda says she feels at a loss to know what to say to him. She says that she wishes they were not together, as she can't handle his feelings as well as her own, and still be strong enough to provide care for Michael.

## Reflective **task**

» What 'losses' can you identify in this example?

» From whose perspective?

When we talk about 'loss' in relation to care-giving, it is important for practitioners to recognise and understand that grief and loss are complex issues and reactions to them are shaped and mediated by culture, gender, age and a myriad of other circumstances; clearly grief and loss are not just related to the death of the cared-for person.

Some writers (for example, Wilson et al, 2016), in attempting to provide a framework or typology to support understanding of this complex area, have categorised grief into three distinct stages, each with its own particular impact on carers. In essence these stages are:

- » anticipatory grief;
- » post-death grief;
- » complicated grief.

Anticipatory grief relates to the feelings of loss and bereavement that occur in advance of death, and may also be experienced by the person who is dying as well as their carer.

Post-death grief, according to Wilson et al (2016), involves three stages: grieving, mourning and healing. When practitioners are working with carers who have been bereaved, it is of course unrealistic to expect them to move neatly through the different stages associated with grief. Grieving can be raw, intense and incredibly painful, both physically and emotionally. The 'stage' of mourning implies that this intense emotion is done with, although for many the reality is quite different, and the notion of healing may for many be patronising and completely unrealistic.

Complicated grief is seen as a more extreme form of extended mourning, a more chronic and heightened state of affairs where there may be an inability to accept that the person has died, and an intense, extreme focus on the loss and memories of the loved one.

Carers' experiences of loss and grief are also closely associated with changing self-identity (Murphy et al, 2016). Orzeck and Silverman (2008) suggest that 'post-caregiving', not just that associated with death of the cared-for person needs to be seen as part of the care-giving 'career' and a notable stage of the life course and identity for carers. For many carers, grief following bereavement may bring about a range of emotions. It obviously involves a change, which many people find challenging. As well as carers missing the physical presence of the person who has died, for many of them their identity and purpose has also gone. Interactions with paid carers or services that supported the cared-for person may cease abruptly.

## Case example

Anne cared for her husband Norman, who had mental health issues – including depression and anxiety – for five years before one day he took his own life when she had gone on a rare visit to the hairdressers. After the funeral, Anne was telephoned once by Norman's key worker from the community mental health team. That was the only contact Anne received from them, despite their making weekly visits to the home over the past four years.

Anne said she not only missed Norman terribly, but that she also missed seeing the workers from the team who had supported her on a weekly basis. Some weeks they had been the only visitors to the house and now, all of a sudden, she was alone. As well as the physical presence of a visitor to the home, Anne particularly missed knowing that someone was 'interested' in her and she also missed the rhythm and familiarity of a Wednesday afternoon visit.

As stated earlier, grief and loss are complex and for many family carers, even though their relative is alive and may be in good physical or emotional health, there may also be a profound sense of loss of what might have been.

For many parents the birth, or diagnosis of a child with a disability is seen as being like meeting a stranger; the child and the expected future is not what was planned. This notion of grief, and those feelings that accompany 'what might have been' has been termed 'chronic sorrow'. It was first noted in 1962 by sociologist Simon Olshansky (Olshansky, 1962, cited in Roos, 2002), who observed that parents of children with what is now known in the UK as learning difficulties, demonstrated periodic and recurrent grief. He believed that the issues of long-term ongoing care-giving burdens were powerful enough to set in motion feelings of chronic sorrow. Grieving for what might have been meant that parents did not ever have 'closure'.

What might have been, what possibilities exist when compared to peers, is difficult for parents to ignore, especially when faced with discrimination and prejudice that is a feature of everyday life for people with disabilities. Segregation and difference mark out the experience of children growing up with a disability and parents have to try and help their offspring (including siblings) make sense of the world, in cases where there seems to be no rational explanation.

Milestones reached often bring with them a reminder of the hopes and plans that have now been changed – some for better, some for worse – but overall difference exists and carers are generally the ones on whom it impacts second (?).

## Case example

Asha's son, Naz, has a severe learning difficulty that was diagnosed shortly after his birth 19 years ago. Naz has some mobility issues; he requires support with his personal care, including feeding and changing. He does not verbalise, uses pictures in order to communicate and attends a specialist education provision 15 miles from the family home. Paid carers visit twice a day to assist Asha with Naz's care.

On a day-to-day basis Asha feels that she manages Naz's care well, and she says she loves him unreservedly, admires his resilience and his overriding sense of fun. Asha is still in touch with friends she made at ante-natal classes, and she says it is these moments that bring about to her the recognition of the stark difference between Naz's life and those of his peers.

Obtaining GSCEs, learning to drive, having a part-time job, and going to university are just some of the moments Asha has celebrated with her friends' children that she has not experienced with Naz. While it is a different life from that she envisaged and she says she wouldn't change a thing, Asha says she still feels an acute sense of loss for what 'might have been'.

Strohm (2004) also describes this enduring level of sadness as chronic. Chronic sorrow is the presence of recurring and ongoing intense feelings of sadness in the lives of carers of children who have disabilities. Olshanskey (1962, cited in Roos, 2002: 1) warned professionals that parents would not just 'get over' the birth or diagnosis of a child with impairment(s); rather the grief experienced would be a living loss. In essence 'chronic sorrow' is response to a loss, described by Roos (2002) as an emotion-filled tension between 'what is' versus the carer's view of 'what should have been'.

## Personal **reflection**

Feelings of 'what might have been' sometimes seem to come from nowhere and when you are least expecting them. A friend of mine who has a child with severe learning difficulties told me how she was interviewing potential students recently for an occupational therapy programme. Glancing at an application from a potential student she noticed that he had the same birthday as her 18-year-old son. She recalled that she struggled to control her emotions; her son, whom she loves immensely, requires 24-hour care and struggles to write his own name and yet, here in front of her, born on the same day, was a confident young man with an impressive range of GCSEs and anticipated high-grade 'A' levels. My friend described to me how she was suddenly transported back to that day, 18 years ago, when her son came into the world; and she thought about the other Mum and the hopes, dreams and aspirations that she imagined they may both have shared for their sons.

Given the statistics that show that one in five of us will become carers one day, and the demographics that indicate this number will rise (Carers UK, 2015), recognising and understanding issues of grief and loss cannot be ignored. For practitioners, as well as contemplating how best to inform their own practice, there is the very real possibility that they also will be the ones either providing or receiving family care in their personal lives, and an acknowledgement of some of the emotions that run alongside that scenario need to be brought into the open. Given the enormity, and likelihood of that scenario for many of us, it would seem to be a question that is worthy of discussion and further exploration.

It is important to develop a deeper understanding of carers' perceptions of grief, loss and bereavement, as this has the potential to help practitioners in a number of ways – to facilitate acknowledgement, greater support and therefore perhaps assist carers to develop greater resilience in the future.

How then might practitioners look to support carers who are bereaved or grieving, whether that is through a death of a person, or an unwanted change in circumstances? The importance of communication cannot be underplayed.

It is important to acknowledge the situation that carers are going through, as well as remembering that carers' grief may trigger many different and unexpected emotions. Feelings of grief and bereavement are natural and individual; what one person experiences and the way they react will not be the same for another. Practitioners working with carers who have been bereaved must remember that the grieving process will be unique to each carer. There is no right or wrong way for carers to grieve. How carers grieve will depend on many factors, including their relationship with the person who has died, their personality and how they deal with stress, as well as what else is going on in their life at the time. Grieving cannot be rushed. There are no short cuts and family carers, like everyone else who has been bereaved and is grieving, need to get through it – there is no going round it. Whichever and however carers experience grief, it is important for others to be patient and acknowledge that it will take time before one begins to feel even a tiny bit better. For carers of people with a terminal illness, it is important that support for those carers focuses not only on supporting practical skills, such as physical tending, but also on supporting carers including acknowledgement of, and preparedness for, the death of the cared-for person.

In 1969, Swiss-American psychiatrist, Elisabeth Kübler-Ross, in her book on death and dying, introduced a theory of grief which became known as the 'five stages of grief'. These stages of grief were based on her studies of the way she believed people felt when approaching death. Over time, these stages have been generalised into other life challenges, including other changes that incorporate loss – for example, a divorce, being made redundant, or a physical life-changing illness or injury. Knowing more about the work of Kübler-Ross is useful for practitioners in terms of developing knowledge and understanding.

In essence the stages referred to by Kübler-Ross (1969) are as follows:

» Denial: This is the 'stage' of disbelief; people may be in shock, may feel completely overwhelmed and numb and wonder how they can carry on at all.

» Anger: This is seen as a necessary 'stage' in the healing process. Questions are asked and accusations made; people may look for someone to blame, and ask questions such as 'Why is this is happening? – Who's fault is this?'

» Bargaining: This relates to requests often considered to be to a higher deity – for example: 'I will do this, if you make this not happen'; or 'I will devote my life to whatever, if you just take this away'.

» Depression: This relates to a feeling of despair, a feeling of being too sad to do anything. The fact remains that the death of a loved one can be a very depressing and sad situation and feelings of depression, as with denial and anger, are natural states of mind.

» Acceptance: The idea of acceptance does not mean that everything is alright and back to 'normal' – rather it equates to being able to function on a day-to-day basis while recognising that things will never be the same again.

For many carers their post-caring life may be felt almost as a betrayal. Now, for example, finally they can go out on a whim and can visit friends, or travel. This may bring with it feelings of guilt as well; well-meaning friends and perhaps health and social care professionals may make comments about a cared-for person's death such as: 'It's for the best' and 'at least you can have your life back now', when it might be that the only thing the carer wants is for the person who has died to be alive.

For many carers, though the loss and grief associated with bereavement is incredibly traumatic, we know that bereavement is associated not only with adverse health effects, but also a higher risk of dying oneself (Stroebe and Schut, 2015).

Dealing with changes, living with uncertainty and transitioning to new roles are all aspects of providing care that family carers may have to deal with throughout their caring 'career'. Timeliness and consistency are needed in offering support post-caring, as is a sensitive and person-centred approach. A recent bereavement may bring up other times of loss, sadness and grief from many years ago, and health and social care practitioners need to be mindful that what they may think of as an insignificant loss, for example, of a part-time job, may be to a carer the final straw and may bring back memories of other more traumatic losses in the past.

# Carers and spirituality

As we noted in Chapter 7, factors affecting the resilience and resourcefulness of carers are complex; however, it may be the case that carers who identify with having a cultural or spiritual belief may suggest that it brings meaning and hope to their situation. A study of informal care-givers of adults with dementia identified participation in religious activities as one element of managing stress and developing resilience (Ross et al, 2003). Having a belief and/or life philosophy has long been recognised as a 'protective factor' in determining both the likelihood of experiencing a stressful situation, but also of having the ability to deal with and adapt to adverse changes. Spirituality may be seen as an internal coping resource to buffer the effects of uncertainty on emotional well-being (Chan et al, 2015), and one that may enable carers to continue when situations become particularly challenging. Spirituality can also be defined as our sense of meaning in life (Mitchell, 2015), and as such, having a spiritual identity relates to the concept of a person's sense of meaning and purpose in life which may, or may not, be expressed through formal religious beliefs and practices. For Greasley et al (2001), the idea of spiritual care within caring situations is associated with the quality of interpersonal care in terms of the expression of love and compassion. For Ahmet and Victor cited in Hjelm, 2015), the evidence base for the role of religion in care and caring is not a robust one. Ethnic minority carers, for example, believe that research does not take account of the importance of religion. Practitioners working with carers need to be sensitive to the unique situations they are in and of cultural, spiritual and religious beliefs and the importance carers and the person in receipt of their care may place upon them, as well as recognising that spirituality may appear to be linked with their resilience.

# Looking to the future: tips for busy practitioners working with carers

I hope that by reading this book, you have found something that has made you think, or (re)consider yours and others' work with carers. It is not easy. The lives and issues faced by carers, like everyone else, can be incredibly complex; situations are diverse, and responses to them vary.

Of course, there is always much more that could be said, especially with such a multi-faceted topic. However, the points highlighted in this book constitute what I believe demonstrates good practice.

The final points relate to practical guidance for practitioners – some you may have heard of, or thought of before, others not – and their applicability to your own situation will vary. They are intended as ways of encouraging you to continue the work you are doing.

## Empathic reflexivity

Reflexivity is currently a dominant model for practice within health care and social work. It is designed to address some of the imbalance of power relations between health and social care workers and the people with whom they work. Most of us will have had the experience of copying someone else's behaviours, subconsciously at times. Think, for example, of a time when you have been in a situation where someone began yawning, or laughing, and you joined in. Have you ever fed a baby, and found yourself opening your own mouth, or swallowing? Taking this one step further and being conscious of what you are doing or – to put it another way – imagine that you are in that person's shoes. What might that feel like? It is not easy. I cannot imagine what it would be like to be a carer for a parent with dementia. However, there are parallels that I can draw on from my experience of working with carers who are in that situation, and my experiences as a parent-carer may offer me some insight into the challenges and rewards of a caring scenario. There are, of course, dangers with that, and pitfalls to be avoided include the transposing of one's own experiences onto other people. Working with people is not rocket science; I would contend it is much more complex. The reactions of humans to an immeasurable range of circumstances, while in some situations may show some similarity, are also unpredictable. You may think that you know exactly how a carer will respond to a given situation based on your own experiences of working with carers and of perhaps being a carer yourself. However, there are no cast iron guarantees.

## Being organised

When you are really busy and struggling to get everything done, as basic as it sounds – write a list. Write down everything you have to do, including deadlines, and then number everything in order of importance. Work your way through the list from most important to least important. I like the idea of moving deadlines earlier, even if only in your head, as that helps to ensure that you have had the 'adrenaline rush' that accompanies the end of a project. Someone I know, who loves to celebrate Christmas, always pretends that it takes place at Thanksgiving (the fourth Thursday in November, which she doesn't celebrate). By then she has bought and wrapped and planned menus and food shopping lists for 25 December. That way she says she is ahead of the game, and can really enjoy the Christmas celebrations. She knows that it is a fact that on 25 December she will celebrate Christmas each year. Her reasoning is that it is not unexpected, so why would you not plan in good time?

If you use a list, be sure to cross things off as you go along, as this will give you a sense of accomplishment, and at the end of each week or month take a moment to look at your list and see just how much you have achieved.

## Seeking advice

Some of the most effective leaders in the world are not afraid to seek advice. For health and social care practitioners, supervision and mentorship are key to successful and longevity of roles. Make use of supervision; go prepared to seek and heed advice; set goals; practise active listening skills; be a lifelong learner; recognise that your work is a long-term investment and that there are no short cuts. Difficult as it sounds, when time is short and activities are pressing, do try to make time to network and meet other people; don't stay isolated in your office. Time attending conferences and training may be seen as a luxury by some, but they do provide you with an opportunity to learn from others, ask questions and consider ways of developing and improving your own skills. Attending live events, such as conferences and training, may be invigorating and yes, they might be expensive for employers, but so too is high staff turnover. New ideas and approaches gained from such events may allow health and social care practitioners to become more effective in what they do, and may increase efficiency.

In terms of working with others, attendance at inter- and multi-disciplinary events, conferences and training can be vital.

Other options to consider as well as attending conferences and external training events are webinars, reading blogs and listening to podcasts. Social networking may be a valuable tool in keeping connected with peers; however, there is little to beat actually meeting and having a face-to-face conversation with someone. Fresh thinking and new ideas are born from being in different environments and meeting different people. To coin an oft-quoted advertising phrase: 'It's because you're worth it' – if you are investing in your work, recognising that you always have things to learn, then surely the recipients of your practice will also benefit?

## Being honest

When working with carers, don't pretend that you know all the answers. If you do not know the answer to a question you have been asked, say so, then go and find out the answer and be sure to get back to the carer and tell them. It is important to keep in touch, even if you haven't yet found the answer to the question. By giving a carer a call and saying you haven't forgotten to check out that service/allowance/group that they asked you about (you may not have had a response from a phone message to someone), then tell the carers that. Carers cannot read your mind, and by you thinking you'll wait until the group leader gets back to you before you get back to the carer (to use what seems like a very long-winded example!), in the carer's mind this means that you have forgotten them and that their situation is unimportant. Far better to leave a quick message saying you are trying to find out, you will keep trying and then will call the carer back in X number of days with an update – and then do so. Be sure to keep a clear record of your workload and what you have to do over the next few weeks. That way, if you are ever ill, or have to leave the office for an emergency, someone else will be able to check your notes and telephone or email on your behalf. We all carry so much information in our heads – by transferring that to paper, or an online diary accessible by others, takes a few more minutes, but is time well spent.

If people know what is going on they are much more likely to be supportive in your efforts and of course, it helps to build your relationship. Most of the complaints about professionals from carers and service users are not to do with lack of services, they are to do with the way that they have been treated – something that you can address.

Take time to read and speak to people; thinking time is severely underrated. You need time to process emotions; try to keep fit. Maintain and sustain other interests, however limited the time might be for them.

## Maintaining a critical gaze

Imagine a film being taken of your relationship and interactions with a carer. Consider for a moment: from which angle would the film shots be taken? Who is in control of the camera and decides when and what to film and when to stop? Would certain elements of the interaction be edited out and left on the cutting-room floor? Whose perspective would be privileged? Imagine that the camera would put the audience into the perspective of the carer. Whose gaze takes precedence in the telling of the story being filmed and how would carers be portrayed from different angles?

This for me in essence is what the notion of a critical gaze is about; attempting to look outside the box and view situations from another angle. One's lived experiences – be that as a practitioner, or as a carer – shape one's existence and accordingly, one's behaviour. Much attention is paid (rightly so) to the importance of adopting an anti-oppressive approach to work in the caring professions. The focus of much of this attention is at a macro-level, for example, policies imposed from the 'top down' of managerial structures and hierarchies. In order for practitioners to develop and maintain a 'critical gaze', it is necessary to examines one's own practice on an individual level. Practitioners must consider the strengths and assets of carers as well as their needs and must be prepared to recognise, acknowledge and challenge the at times inhuman structures of society, as well as recognising, acknowledging, and challenging the unequal power direction between themselves and carers and the people who are supported by carers.

Adopting a critical gaze may provide momentum and confidence for practitioners to challenge any instances of power imbalance or oppressive experiences they observe, or are party to. Techniques to support this include individuals taking responsibility and being clear about the responsibility of others, and a focus on meaningful discourse and empowerment, brought about by reflexive empathy.

## Being clear about what you mean

For practitioners with responsibility for completing and recording carers' needs, assessments need to be clear about what they are recording and who said it. The complexity of any caring situation is unlikely to be captured in a few words or lines. For example, reading in a carer's assessment: 'Mrs S supports son with bathing and medication' may in no way reflect the complexity of those acts. Think about the challenge of encouraging someone to have a bath when they don't want one. For example, a parent with a teenage son who has severe learning difficulties and who has smeared faeces over the bathroom wall, and all over himself, will clearly need a bath or a shower. The same teenage son may be 6ft (182cm) tall and weigh 16 stone (101.6kg) – and no way does he see the need for a shower. Think about that for a moment – what do you think a carer would do?

Likewise 'supports with medication' may conjure up an image of a couple of tablets being dispensed into a willing and grateful spouse's hand. The reality may be that the same spouse has dementia, and is convinced you are trying to poison him/her. Eye drops also need to be administered, and yet they refuse to open their eyes.

To record these activities as 'support with bathing and medication' may not resemble the reality of the experience for many carers. Being clear and providing such details in an assessment may help to obtain services, or ensure that referrals are accepted by other organisations, and this alone may have a substantial effect on the lives and well-being of carers and of those they support. A skilled practitioner may be able to elicit the reality from some carers, although of course this is not guaranteed.

Prior to the introduction of the Care Act (2014) carers did not have the same entitlement to assessment and services as people in receipt of care. However, the importance of carers and the recognition of the important role they play in health and social care does now appear to be becoming recognised in some areas; there is still a long way to go. Given the current financial crisis, cuts to services and a period of austerity where everyone is expected to do more with less, I contend this includes practitioners as well as carers and people with care and support needs. Being creative and resourceful, combined with carrying out relevant and timely research may provide dividends for all in the longer term. In spite of this, I do believe that practitioners might have all the skills, knowledge, experience and understanding in the world, but in order to do what they need to do best to support carers, as well as those people with care and support needs, they will need more than that. What is needed are resources – lots of them. Research reports continue to indicate that the system of care in the UK is under-resourced, and that new policy measures are called for. Although, as noted elsewhere, legislation relating to care has been reformed, implementation of the Care Act (2014) and associated legislation falls on local authorities, who are operating a reduced service in the light of cuts to their own services and other austerity measures.

Practitioners' creativity, excellent communication skills and empathy go a long way to supporting carers without significant additional resources. However, without access to additional services – be that help in the home, or externally – the limitations placed on carers by the lack of appropriate, affordable, flexible services to meet the needs of the person being cared for, *as well as* for family carers, the pressures they experience will remain. Raising awareness of carers' issues, campaigning and spreading the word, while not necessarily made explicit in practitioners' job descriptions, might go some way to help society to recognise the existence and the needs of carers. Carers do the best they can do with what they have access to. You could make a (big) difference, not just for them but for the people who rely upon them.

## Taking it further

1. Safeguarding is a complex issue; for further information please see the following sources:

    NHS England. *Safeguarding Vulnerable People in the NHS – Accountability and Assurance Framework*, www.england.nhs.uk/wp-content/uploads/2015/07/safeguarding-accountability-assurance-framework.pdf.

2. For issues of loss and grief see J. Hefel, Will you be with me to the end?, in Witkin, S L (ed) (2014) *Narrating Social Work through Auto-Ethnography*, ch. 8. New York: Columbia University Press. This source uses auto-ethnography, an innovative approach to inquiry, to discuss this personal issue.

# References

Atkinson, S, Fuller, S and Painter, J (2016) *Wellbeing and Place*. London: Routledge.

Camic, P M and Chatterjee, H J (2013) Museums and art galleries as partners for public health interventions. *Perspectives in Public Health*, *133*(1): 66–71.

Carers UK (2015) *Valuing Carers 2015 – the Rising Value of Carers' Support*. University of Sheffield, University of Leeds and CIRCLE: Carers UK.

Chan, K P C, Lo, H Y P and Ho, R T H (2015) Spirituality in family care-giving of schizophrenia: the role of attachment to divinity. Paper presented at the *Annual Meeting and Scientific Sessions of the Society of Behavioral Medicine, SBM 2015*, held San Antonio, Texas, 22–25 April 2015.

Cooney, C, Howard, R and Lawlor, B (2006) Abuse of vulnerable people with dementia by their carers: can we identify those most at risk? *International Journal of Geriatric Psychiatry*, *21*(6): 564–71.

Cooper, S A, Smiley, E, Jackson, A, Finlayson, J, Allan, L, Mantry, D and Morrison, J (2009) Adults with intellectual disabilities: prevalence, incidence and remission of aggressive behaviour and related factors. *Journal of Intellectual Disability Research*, *53*(3): 217–32.

Dodd, J (2002) Museums and the health of the community. In *Museums, Society, Inequality* (pp 182–9). London: Routledge.

Feldon, P (2017) *The Social Worker's Guide to the Care Act 2014*. St Albans: Critical Publishing.

Greasley, P, Chiu, L F and Gartland, R M (2001) The concept of spiritual care in mental health nursing. *Journal of Advanced Nursing*, *33*(5): 629–37.

Hjelm, T (ed) (2015) *Is God Back? Reconsidering the New Visibility of Religion*. London: Bloomsbury.

HM Government (2011) No health without mental health. www.gov.uk/government/uploads/system/uploads/attachment_data/file/213761/dh_124058.pdf [accessed 29 March 2018].

Holt, A (2016) Adolescent-to-parent abuse as a form of 'domestic violence': a conceptual review. *Trauma, Violence, & Abuse*, *17*(5): 490–9.

Kleinman, A (2012) Caregiving as moral experience. *The Lancet*, *380*(9853): 1550–51.

Kübler-Ross, E (2003 [1969]) *On Death and Dying*. New York: Scribner Classics.

Marriott, H (2003) *The Selfish Pig's Guide to Caring*. Clifton-upon-Teme: Polperro Heritage Press.

Mitchell, D (2015) Spiritual and cultural issues at the end of life. *Medicine*, *43*(12): 740–1.

Murphy, G, Peters, K, Wilkes, L M and Jackson, D (2016) Adult children of parents with mental illness: losing oneself. Who am I? *Issues in Mental Health Nursing*, *37*(9): 668–73.

Orzeck, P and Silverman, M (2008) Recognizing post-caregiving as part of the caregiving career: implications for practice. *Journal of Social Work Practice*, *22*(2): 211–20.

Roberts, S, Camic, P M and Springham, N (2011) New roles for art galleries: art-viewing as a community intervention for family carers of people with mental health problems. *Arts & Health*, *3*(2): 146–59.

Roos, S (2002) *Chronic Sorrow: A Living Loss*. Hove: Psychology Press.

Ross, L, Holliman, D and Dixon, D R (2003) Resiliency in family care-givers: implications for social work practice. *Journal of Gerontological Social Work*, *40*(3): 81–96.

Selwood, A, Cooper, C, Owens, C, Blanchard, M and Livingston, G (2009) What would help me stop abusing? The family carer's perspective. *International Psychogeriatrics*, *21*(2): 309–13.

Stroebe, M and Schut, H (2015) Family matters in bereavement: toward an integrative intra-interpersonal coping model. *Perspectives on Psychological Science*, *10*(6): 873–9.

Strohm, K (2004) *Siblings: Coming Unstuck and Putting Back the Pieces*. London: David Fulton.

Tyrer, F, McGrother, C W, Thorp, C F, Donaldson, M, Bhaumik, S, Watson, J M and Hollin, C (2006) Physical aggression towards others in adults with learning disabilities: prevalence and associated factors. *Journal of Intellectual Disability Research*, *50*(4): 295–304.

Vaddadi, K S, Gilleard, C and Fryer, H (2002) Abuse of carers by relatives with severe mental illness. *International Journal of Social Psychiatry*, *48*(2): 149–55.

Walsh, J A and Krienert, J L (2007) Child–parent violence: an empirical analysis of offender, victim, and event characteristics in a national sample of reported incidents. *Journal of Family Violence*, *22*(7): 563–74.

Walsh, S M, Martin, S C and Schmidt, L A (2004) Testing the efficacy of a creative-arts intervention with family caregivers of patients with cancer. *Journal of Nursing Scholarship*, *36*(3): 214–19.

Wilson, S, Toye, C, Aoun, S, Slatyer, S, Moyle, W and Beattie, E (2016) Effectiveness of psychosocial interventions in reducing grief experienced by family carers of people with dementia: a systematic review protocol. *JBI Database of Systematic Reviews and Implementation Reports*, *14*(6): 30–41.

Yan, E (2014) Abuse of older persons with dementia by family caregivers: results of a 6-month prospective study in Hong Kong. *International Journal of Geriatric Psychiatry*, *29*(10): 1018–27.

# Index

acceptance, in grief, 164
Adams, J, 126
ADASS. *See* Association of Directors of Adult Social Services
Alzheimer's dementia, 146
anger, in grief, 164
anticipatory grief, 160
Asian carers, 34
assessed and supported year of employment (ASYE), 88
assessments, 50
  case study, 98
  role for practitioners, 97–98
Association of Carers, 22
Association of Directors of Adult Social Services (ADASS), 43
ASYE. *See* assessed and supported year of employment
Atkin, K, 15, 85, 92
Attendance Allowance, 38
austerity, 60, 76

baby care, 78–80
Bangladeshi carers, 34
bargaining, in grief, 164
BASW. *See* British Association of Social Workers
Becker, S, 133
Beveridge, W, 43, 48
British Association of Social Workers (BASW), 116
Butler Act, 43

care
  community, 27–30
  definition of, 4
  dynamics of, 9
  ethical and political dimensions, 14
  ethical debates, 118–119
  impact of, 30–31
  neoliberalism, 47
  partners in, 85–88
  reciprocal, 33
  reflective task, 20
  short break, 80–82

Care Act 2014, 3, 15, 24, 49, 50, 70, 81, 85, 93, 124, 133, 152
  section 42 of, 153–154
  section 44 of, 155
Care and Support Statutory Guidance, 50, 101, 102
Care Bill, 85
care in institutions, 27–30
care-giver, definition of, 4
care-giving
  dynamics of, 9
  emotional and psychological challenges of, 1
  implications of, 14
carer. *See also* professional carers, young carer
  abusive behaviour, 148
  and choice, 54–55
  as co-clients, 93
  as co-worker, 92, 93
  as resource, 92, 93
  as superseded, 94
  cards/passports, 156
  case study, 64–65
  change in identity, 76–78
  choice as positive entity, 55–56
  community on, 30–31
  daily living, 66–68
  definition of, 5
  emergency cards, 156
  employment and, 56–59
  family, 25, 31, 148
  frustrations, 69
  history and development of organisations, policy and legislation, 26
  impact on, 11
  individual budget for, 51–52
  knowledge, 11
  non-carer and, 67
  partnership working, 86
  political ideologies, 45–46
  practitioners working with, 158
  professional. *See* professional carers
  resilient, 122
  respite, 80–82

carer. *See also* professional carers,
    young carer (*cont.*)
  rights vs disabled people's rights, 32–35
  shame/guilt, 77
  skills, 11
  social policy, 49–51
  spirituality and, 165–166
  stress, 64, 68–71
  students as, 139–140
  values of, 12
care-receiver, 10
Carer's Allowance, 73
carer's assessments
  beginning assessment, 100
  combined assessments, 101–106
  stages of, 99
Carers National Association, 23
Carers (Recognition and Services) Act 1995,
    49, 131
Carers Trust, 19, 23, 57, 140
Carers UK, 19, 31, 54, 135
caring
  for and about, 8
  for children and babies, 78–80
  gender balance and age, 37
  gender differences, 35–36
  metaphysics of, 16
  positive experience, 119–120
  socio-political ideologies, 76
  Twigg and Atkin's model of, 92–95
caring for adults with dementia, 146–149
Census 2001, 25
Census data, 44–45
Cherry, M G, 77
Children Act 1948, 43
Children and Families Act 2014, 50, 133
children care, 78–80
Chiu, L F, 165
choice carers, 54–55
chronic sorrow, 161, 162
Clements, L J, 33, 35
client group, 92
Cockburn, P, 29
collaborative working, 89
collectivism, 48
combined assessments, 70, 101–106
community care, 27–30
community on carers, 30–31
complicated grief, 160
Crane, N, 23

critical social work practice, 4
Crossroads Care, 23

daily living, carer, 66–68
dementia, 146
denial, in grief, 164
depression, in grief, 164
deprivation of intimate exchange, 68
deprivation of liberty, 29
digital literacy, 116
Dillenburger, K, 117
disabled people's rights vs carers'
    rights, 32–35
DoL. *See* deprivation of liberty

Economic and Social Research Council
    (ESRC)
  description of, 113
  priorities of, 113
Education Act 1944, 43
egalitarianism, 48
Emerson, E, 142
empathic reflexivity, 166
employment, carers and, 56–59
ESRC. *See* Economic and Social Research
    Council
ethics of care, 15, 108, 118–119
European Union, 55

Family Allowances Act 1945, 43
family carers, 25, 31, 73, 148
  collectivism, 48
  legislation and, 42
Feldon, P, 102
financial interdependence, 34
Finch, J, 28
Fine, M, 145
Flexner, A, 95
Foster, L, 56

Gartland, R M, 165
gender
  balance and age, 37
  differences in caring, 35–36
George, V, 46
Gilligan, C, 119
Glendinning, C, 145
Greasley, P, 165
grief
  categories of, 160

stages of, 164
grieving, 161, 164

Hatton, C, 142
HCPC. *See* Health and Care Professions Council
Health and Care Professions Council (HCPC), 120
health and social care practitioners, 11, 110
Heller, T, 33
Heywood, A, 46
Hothersall, S J, 41, 45

identity of carers, 71
ideology
    definition of, 46
    interpretation of, 45
    political, 45–46
imposter syndrome, 91
informal care, 92
informal caring networks, 31
interdependence, 34
inter-professional working, 4, 89

Jones, S, 69

Kleinman, A, 16, 152
knowledge of carers, 11
Kübler-Ross, E, 164

law
    comprehensive understanding of, 41
    definition of, 41
Leu, A, 133
liberal democracy, 46
local authority, 11, 153

McKerr, L, 117
Marriot, H, 158
Maslow, 6
Maslow's hierarchy of need, 6
Meghji, S, 79
Mental Capacity Act, 29
Mental Incapacity Act, 28
meta-ideology of carers, 46
mixed-methods research (MMR), 110
MMR. *See* mixed-methods research
Mockford, C, 117
Morris, J, 32, 33
multi-professional working, 89

National Assistance Act 1948, 43
National Council for Carers and their Elderly Dependents (NCCED), 22
National Council for the Single Woman and her Dependents (NCSWD), 22, 43
National Health Service Act 1946, 43
National Health Service and Community Care Act (NHSCCA), 27
National Insurance (Industrial Injuries) Act 1946, 43
National Insurance Act 1946, 43
NCCED. *See* National Council for Carers and their Elderly Dependents
NCSWD. *See* National Council for the Single Woman and her Dependents
neoliberalism
    care and, 47
    case example, 48
    collectivism, 48
    definition of, 46
    egalitarianism, 48
NHSCCA. *See* National Health Service and Community Care Act
non-carers, 67

Office for National Statistics (ONS), 131
older parent carer
    case example, 143
    challenges, 142
    dependent relationship, 143
    description of, 141
    experiences of, 143
    financial issues, 144
    for practitioners, 145
    misunderstandings, 141
    practical, physical and emotional care, 142
    reciprocity issues, 146
    throwaway comment, 141
Olshansky, S, 161, 162
ONS. *See* Office for National Statistics
Orzeck, P, 160
Oxenham, M F, 19, 20

*P v Cheshire West and Chester Council*, 30
*P&Q v Surrey County Council*, 30
partners in care, 85–88
partnership working, 86
Pearlin, L I, 68
personalisation, 51–52
political ideologies of carers, 45–46

post-caring
    anticipatory grief, 160
    case examples, 159, 161, 162
    complicated grief, 160
    loss and grief, 158
    post-death grief, 160
post-death grief, 160
practice-based research, 118
practitioner, 11
    implications for, 60
    in assessments, 97–98
    resilience of, 125
    toolkit, 75
practitioner guidance for carers
    being clear, 169–170
    being honest, 168
    being organized, 167
    critical gaze, 169
    empathic reflexivity, 166
    seeking advice, 167–168
Princess Royal Trust for Carers, 23
professional carers
    description of, 89–91
    imposter syndrome, 91
professional resilience, 121, 125–126
professionalism, 95
professionals
    core values, 97
    definition of, 95
Pryce, C, 79

reciprocal care, 33
reflexivity, 166
relational deprivation, 68
research
    characteristics of carer, 116
    definition of, 108
    health and social care, 109
    in social media, 115–118
    language of, 109
research inquiry, 110
research methodology, 109
resilience
    case example, 124
    concept of, 120
    internal characteristics, 122
    literature on, 122
    of practitioners, 125
    professional, 121, 125–126
resilient carer, 122

respite care, 80–82
Robinson, C, 69
Roman Charity, 20
Roos, S, 162
Russell, D P, 85

SAB. See Safeguarding Adults Board
safeguarding
    description of, 152
    principles, 153
    section 42 of Care Act 2014, 153–154
Safeguarding Adults Board (SAB), 154
Safeguarding Adults Review (SAR), 155–158
safeguarding vulnerable groups, 4
SAR. See Safeguarding Adults Review
self-care, 126
severe learning disability, 4
Sheard, A, 126
short break care, 80–82
Silent Minority (documentary film), 28
Silverman, M, 160
skills of carers, 11
sleep deprivation, 66
small-scale community initiatives, 47
social capital, 157
Social Care Institute for Excellence, 103
social liberalism, 46
social media, 115–118
social policy, 49–51
social revolution, 22
social welfare reform, 47
social work law and ethics, 4
social worker, 3
spirituality, 165–166
statute law, 41
stress, carer, 68–71
Strohm, K, 162
student dissertations, 114
students as carers, 139–140
sustainability, 103

Taylor, S E, 36
Thatcher, M, 27
Thomas, N, 134
Thomson, C, 58
Tilley, L, 19, 20
Todd, S, 69
Tronto, J, 56
Twigg and Atkin's model of caring, 92–95
Twigg, J, 15, 85, 92